A Personal Essay on the History of Neonatal Nursing

Looking Back to See the Road Ahead

Kaye Spence AM
2022

First published by Busybird Publishing 2022

Copyright © 2022 Kathryn Kaye Spence AM

ISBN
Paperback: 978-1-922691-81-1
Ebook: 978-1-922691-82-8

This work is copyright. Apart from any use permitted under the *Copyright Act 1968*, no part of this publication may be reproduced, stored in a retrieval system or transmitted in any form or by any means, electronic, mechanical, photocopying, recording or otherwise, without the prior written permission of Kathryn Kaye Spence AM.

The information in this book is based on the author's experiences and opinions. The author and publisher disclaim responsibility for any adverse consequences, which may result from use of the information contained herein. Permission to use any external content has been sought by the author. Any breaches will be rectified in further editions of the book.

Cover Image: Supplied by the Author

Cover design: Busybird Publishing

Layout and typesetting: Busybird Publishing

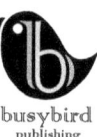

Busybird Publishing
2/118 Para Road
Montmorency, Victoria
Australia 3094
www.busybird.com.au

Author

Kaye Spence AM has been a neonatal nurse for over 45 years. Kaye has worked in Sydney, London, and the Gold Coast, Queensland. She holds an honorary position as Adjunct Associate Professor at Western Sydney University and is a Clinical Nurse Consultant in Neonatology at the Royal Alexandra Hospital for Children /The Children's Hospital at Westmead. Kaye is widely published with over 50 publications in textbooks and peer-reviewed journals. Her latest venture is in creative writing, and she has just completed her first novel. She looks forward to pursuing her interests.

http://kathrynkaye.com.au

To: Edward who supported my career, and to the neonatal nurses who inspired my career

Prologue

Passions are activities that you enjoy, that drive you to success and give you satisfaction. Nursing was my passion. As I gained experience with nursing, neonatal nursing became my driving passion. Most employers want to know what inspires and motivates their workforce. What drives them to achieve the goals set by the organisation. Everyone knew my passion. My nursing journey wasn't easy, but I knew this was the path I wanted to take.

I am now working out my last few months of being employed as a neonatal nurse. Good heavens, am I thinking of retirement? This was a word I have avoided and a concept that I struggle to define. I am motivated by the enthusiastic young nurses who now are my colleagues and who inspired me to reflect on my journey through neonatal nursing. Their questions have enabled me to consider the noteworthy events which had an impact on me and the formation of neonatal nursing in New South Wales, across Australia, and into the international community.

It is to those young women that I dedicate this book.

This book is written as a personal essay as I reflect on the history of neonatal nursing in Australia. I have lived this history. Like any reflection, involves memory, my memory is where I keep the information. I have gathered over time information that has influenced my future actions and become a valuable tool. The memories in this book are my memories. Where I have quoted times and years, those details have been supplemented by diary notes I was luckily enough to keep and find.

I have used the names of those influential people in my neonatal journey, and I am sure others may benefit from knowing the names of these pioneers. Other notable names may not occur, and this is because they did not have an impact on my journey and history of neonatal nursing, or I simply forgot.

Like any history there are facts. I have included those that are relevant to my story.

I have had the privilege of living the history of neonatal nursing, especially in New South Wales and across Australia as it became an established sub-specialty in both medicine and nursing. The international communities and specific people have been instrumental and enabled me to keep a global perspective, while Australia played a significant role.

So, as I look to the road ahead, I have found looking back has given me the courage to make that final leap into retirement. I am leaving a profession that has fulfilled me for over 50 years and a specialty that was driven by a passion for newborn infants and their families. We aimed to make those early times spent in the hospital bearable and to give the babies the best possible start in life.

I acknowledge the contribution of Toni Joyce, Julie McNall, and Fiona Wade who have helped me clarify my manuscript. Your edits, thoughts and suggestions were welcome and very much appreciated.

This book is aimed at an audience of neonatal nurses and others with an interest in nursing, both in Australia and internationally. I hope you the reader enjoy these essays and can relate to my experiences as though they are your own.

Kaye Spence AM

Contents

Essay One
Becoming a nurse — 1

Essay Two
Neonatal nursing: change and challenges — 9

Essay Three
Early Days of Learning — 27

Essay Four
Transporting babies: on the road to advanced practice — 37

Essay Five
Pioneers of neonatal nursing — 43

Essay Six
What I have learned from babies — 49

Essay Seven
What I have learned from nurses — 55

Essay Eight
The birth of a professional organisation — 61

Essay Nine
The international stage — 73

Essay Ten
Researching and publishing — 85

Essay Eleven
Those who influenced me — 91

Essay Twelve
A crystal ball to the future — 99

Epilogue — 103

Essay One

Becoming a nurse

I always knew I would become a nurse, at least that is what my mother told me. Evidently, when I was small, (I cannot recall how small), I watched my grandfather in Coffs Harbour prepare a chicken for Sunday lunch. As he chopped off the head, the chicken raced around the yard in a ritualistic dance.

'Look at all the pretty colours coming out of chooky.' I was heard to say.

My mother told me years later that she knew then I was destined to be a nurse. However, this destiny was met with many challenges, some of which I share as they were a significant part of my story.

My passion to become a nurse remained throughout my childhood. I was about eight years old when I visited my twin sister in hospital after her appendix was removed, I went home and carefully cut open my rag doll and removed her 'appendix'. I so impressed everyone with my neat sutures and dressings, I was given a little golden book – Nurse Nancy. This became my bible and, along with the three band-aids stuck inside the front cover, I took to task on anything that needed my attention. I always knew I was going to be a nurse when I grew up. I took subjects in high school such as biology, maths, and English that would be essential for a career in nursing.

However, as we go through life there are always obstacles. When I graduated from school with the Leaving Certificate, the world was my oyster. I applied to the Mater Hospital in Crows Nest in Sydney to begin my training as a nurse. Why did I choose this austere hospital with its army of white-clad nuns? Well, I was born there and felt that must account for something. In addition, one of the nurses who attended my birth, Nona, had become a good friend of my mother. She was my sponsor at my Holy Communion, a sacred event for a young Catholic girl. Those were the days when religion had a spell over me - later it became lost over the years. Nursing is often compared to religion through caring and devotion, as well as the military through the hierarchy and rules. Despite this I was enthusiastic about entering this noble profession, I wanted to be a nurse.

In the mid-1960s I was determined to be independent and have the job I wanted. Remember, this was the time at the beginning of female freedom and people such as Germaine Greer were having an influence on the young women of the time. Not that I knew much about her, only what other girls were saying about the power and influence women can achieve. These were the early days of feminism. With these thoughts, I headed off to my first interview full of confidence that I was going to start my nurse training. Well, I mentioned obstacles before, and I hit one head-on. The Medical Superintendent. These days I look back and wonder what the Medical Superintendent was doing interviewing young women on their own, for a career in nursing. It showed the dominance that the medical profession had over nursing, a dominance that continued for decades. I can still hear his clipped words: -

> *'You have orthostatic albuminuria and would never be strong enough to complete four years of training.'*

I was devastated, I was stopped even before I started. I asked him to let me try and was met with a resounding 'No'. As I look back over 50 years of continuous work as a nurse with years of accumulated sick leave, I would love the opportunity to rub those words in his face! Having confronted one obstacle, little did I know another was to come. My second interview at a prestigious hospital in

Sydney's north was again unsuccessful. This time it was because I was not considered well enough connected with the medical profession, despite my grandfather being a doctor. All the other young women who were interviewed had their fathers, who were doctors, attending the interviews with them. Not a balanced playing field for a young woman with a passion. The great divide had reared its head again, I believed we were all equal. Maybe my naivety allowed me to be blinded to the facts. Now as I look back at the varied backgrounds of the young nurses, I wonder if they had the support of their doctor-fathers?

Someone, (I can't remember who) suggested I try my local hospital. I was still determined to be a nurse and success finally came when I called my local hospital and spoke to the Matron. It turned out to be the best decision I could have made at the time. Ryde District Soldiers Memorial Hospital, unlike the other hospitals, was a small cottage hospital that served the local community of Eastwood, Ryde, and Epping in Sydney My unconventional informal interview was with Matron Lindsay, a motherly character who asked me if I could start the following week. She knew potential at first sight! I was ecstatic - I was going to be a nurse. The four years I spent there were wonderful, full of new experiences and new friends. I learned so much and gained a good broad experience typical of a small hospital, and these experiences have held me strong to this day. The friendships I made then are still friends today.

I donned the starched blue uniform with white collar and cuffs, a crisp white cap, with one embroidered blue pip signifying a first-year cadet, the bright red woollen cape, and my brown lace-up shoes and my career as a nurse started. When I consider the various uniforms, I have worn, they show how nursing has changed, or more specifically how society has influenced the profession. The scrubs nurses wear today are neither professional nor flattering and I thank the lucky stars I have never worn one, except of course when I rotated to work in the operating theatre. When I saw nurses in scrubs pushing trolleys around supermarkets, I felt ashamed. Where have the standards gone? Some even had their names embroidered on their shoulders!

The regimentation and tradition of nursing were part of my training, the archaic practices that seem inconceivable today. We were up at 5.30 am and started our shifts at 6 am. The day began with the ritual of patient baths and sponges; my first patients were the young men whose beds were on the veranda of Ward 2. They all had broken legs following motorbike accidents and they initiated me into the world of caring and being able to laugh at a joke, often at my experience. After one hour on duty, the nurses went to breakfast. During the half-hour meal break, we ate breakfast in the dining room and went to our room where we had to iron our uniforms, polish our shoes, and make our beds before returning promptly to our allocated wards. No wonder I eat fast today as the habit has never left me. Sharing time with others in the nurses' home sealed friendships and I must say improved my cooking skills. We socialised together, explored local haunts, shared stories of new boyfriends, and sometimes we shared boyfriends. There was something about nursing that drew women together and bonded them for life. My best friends were made during those years, friendships that have remained for over 50 years. Louise and I became firm friends almost inseparable. She lives in Toronto, Canada now and has done so for the last 40 years. When we meet up, it is as if the intervening years just fall away, a characteristic of a loyal friend. I think young nurses of today miss this opportunity as the nurses' homes are no longer and those early friendships take a different focus. Many of the new graduate nurses are married and come with a family who support them in their early career, not quite the same as those intimate girlfriends living in the nurses' home.

When I graduated from Ryde after three years and nine months of training (I was in the first group where the four years of training were gradually reduced to three) I was so proud. My last training ward was Ward 6 – paediatrics and I knew this was where my future would be. I loved caring for these little patients and remember I spent my 21st birthday on this ward. I still have the paper silver key and card they made for me. Maybe this was significant – the key to my future.

Despite the obstacles I faced to become a nurse, I believed if you have the passion and the determination you can achieve your goals and in my case my passion. Did my destiny lie in a specific form of nursing? Together with two friends called Carol and Carole, who I had spent the last four years with during our training, we decided to undertake our midwifery training. Off we went to Southport Hospital on the Gold Coast in Queensland to learn about pregnancy, birth, and newborn care. This year provided me with the foundation for my training as a midwife, and I had the pleasure and honour of delivering the required 50 babies. I was exposed to a new world of newly born infants and had a thirst to learn more.

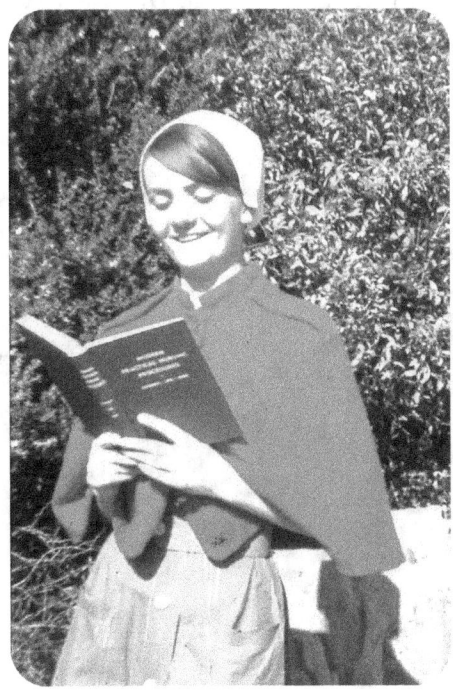

1965 - Kaye in PTS (Preliminary Training School) reading my first textbook - Modern Practical Nursing Procedures by Doherty, Sirl, and Ring. 10th Edition 1963. The Bible so to speak.

To quote from the Preface of this book written by Bruce Mayes, Professor of Obstetrics, University of Sydney.

"The nursing manual marks the end of one epoch and the beginning of another – the end of chaos and the beginning of order. It is a happy coincidence that this work should appear at a time when efforts, unprecedented in our history, are being made to improve the status of the nurse." 1943.

Followed by.

"On its pages may be found clearly and concisely set out the principles governing the practical work that all nurses have to learn, and which they usually acquire during a long and extensive training." R Kirkcaldie, Matron, Royal Alexandra Hospital for Children. 1943

As I read the forty-four chapters, what struck me was how task-orientated this manual was, yet as I flipped through the yellowed pages hidden under these uninspiring headings were the words that eventually guided my practice.

"The prognosis of life for the premature baby depends on – nursing care."

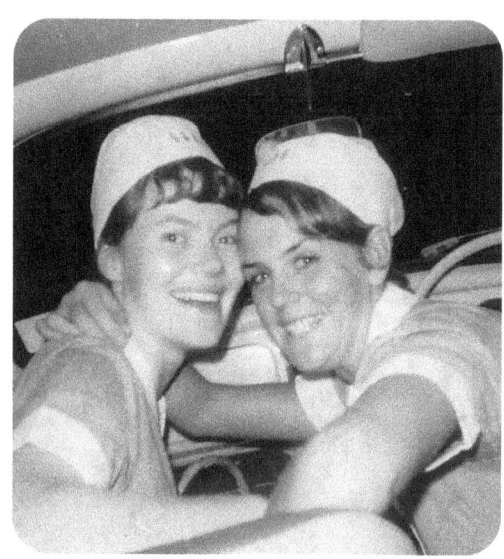

1968 Jackie and Louise – Friends

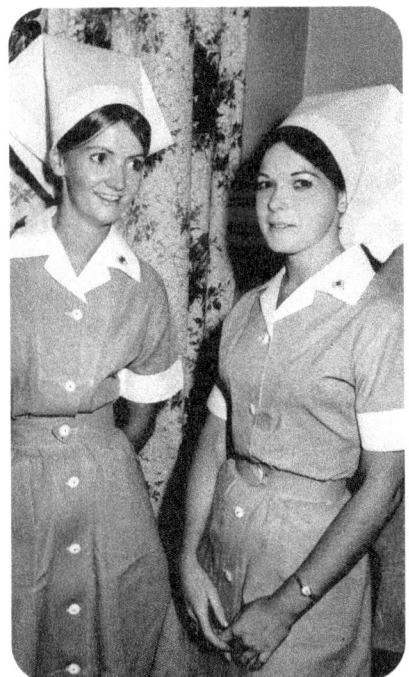

1968 Graduation – Kaye and Carol - Friends

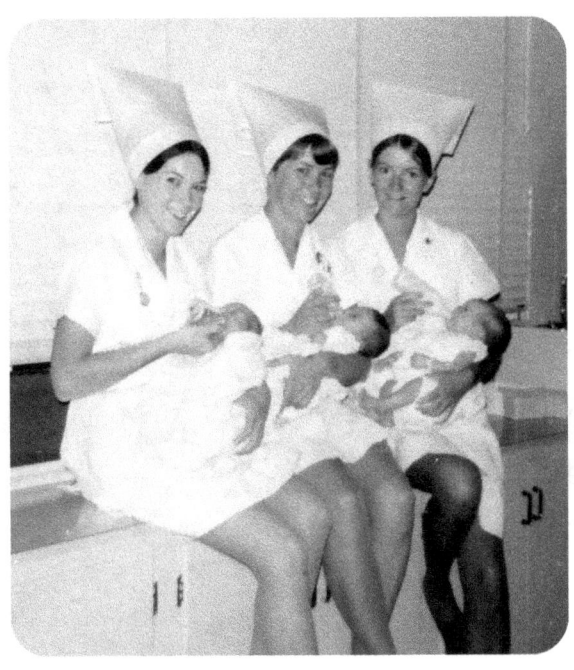

1969 Midwifery at Southport, Queensland – Carol, Dottie, and Kaye

Essay Two

Neonatal nursing: change and challenges

I knew I wanted to take care of babies, especially those who were small, vulnerable, and needing extra care. I graduated as a midwife and then went into paediatrics to become a paediatric nurse, and while babies featured in both these specialties, it was not enough. I wanted to learn more about sick newborns, or neonates. A friend from my general nursing days had premature twin girls born around 28 weeks gestation, which is six months since conception or three months early. The babies were transferred to the Royal Alexandra Hospital for Children in Camperdown where I was working in paediatrics at the time. I was horrified when told that there was nothing that could be done for them, they were too small. I stood looking at these small crimpled red fragile little beings lying in humidicribs struggling to breathe with cold oxygen blasted onto their tiny faces through green rubber funnels. I remember thinking there must be something that could be done for them. They died a few days later after a short and tortuous battle to hold onto life. The year was 1971.

It was during my Paediatric Nursing six-month course that I was introduced to the amazing information that influenced my career. The work of Donald Winnicott (English Paediatrician and Psychoanalyst) who described the importance of a supportive environment for infants and their parents, this information was instrumental to my career. I remembered Jackie's twins and the events of the early 1970s and my determination for a career in neonatal nursing was sealed.

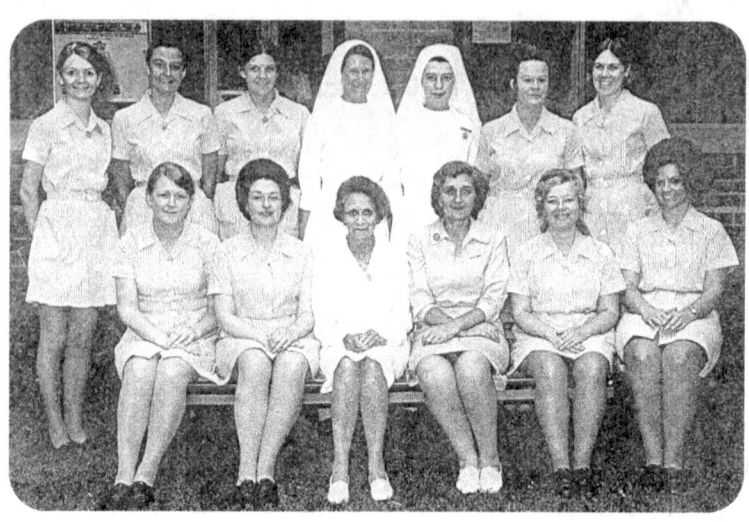

1972 – The first Paediatric Course held at Royal Alexandra Hospital for Children, Camperdown, Sydney. Kaye back row on left, note mini-skirted uniform.

I headed to London to fulfill an ambition to travel around Europe. I took the opportunity to travel by ship, five long, fascinating weeks on board the Fairstair headed for Southampton. I met a lot of people including the ship's nurse, at the time I asked myself why I didn't apply to work my way over as a ship's nurse. It would have saved me the fare but then I would not have had such a great social life on board. When I arrived in London I knew I wanted to gain more experience in nursing as well as travelling. I applied to the prestigious University College Hospital in London and in 1976 I gained a place in their respected neonatal course following a cancellation. My luck changed. This experience was exceptional and was at a time when science was finally helping those babies born prematurely. The early clinical trials of artificial surfactant to minimise respiratory distress syndrome had started. (This was exciting but unfortunately too late to help the twins.)

I was at the cutting edge of science making a major impact on neonatal care, I found this to be both stimulating and rewarding. In London, I had the experience of working with the best, Osmund Reynolds and Jonathan Shaw, two neonatologists together with the influential and pioneer neonatal nurse, Anthea Blake. They shared their varied knowledge and their expertise when they taught us in the neonatal nursing course with openness and genuine interest in debate and questioning. They taught me so much which kept me focussed for over 40 years. I was inspired by these early forerunners, and I believe my life-long contributions to neonatal care stemmed from the influence of those early teachers.

At this time in the mid to late 70s neonatal care was going through a phase of rapid development with clinical trials and new therapies were introduced. I learned about randomised controlled trials and the importance of blind allocation of the patient to the study. I must admit that I and other nurses would hold the opaque envelopes to the light to try to guess who would be allocated into the arm of a trial of the new drug in the Pancuronium trials. As nurses, we all wanted to care for the babies in the experimental arm of the study. Years later, when I was working at the Royal Alexandra Hospital for Children, Camperdown where the NEC trial took place, this same practice remained. Nurses were curious beings! Participating in clinical research was an excellent way to learn and to be able to contribute to developing evidence for practice. The intervention in these studies was harsh and pain and stress were not openly considered. My research interest stemmed from these early experiences and the suffering I saw in these babies.

During three years at University College Hospital in London, I had the opportunity to attend clinics run by Dr. Ann Stewart, a developmental paediatrician whose interest was to measure the outcomes of the babies who had survived newborn intensive care. This was a new area and I remember a discussion we had about how we could improve quality survival by having educated nurses. So now, over 40 years on, we are still having these discussions and undertaking research to show that trained educated nurses can make a difference. Change can be a slow process and shows the uphill battle nurses have had to prove their worth in the emerging scientific and technological environment of health care.

Babies who needed intensive care in the mid-70s often suffered due to the consequences of the treatment as much of it was experimental, and we did what we could as best practice at that time. James (I still remember his name) was a baby I cared for in London over multiple shifts stretching into days and months. He was ventilated for weeks due to his prematurity which resulted in him having sub-glottic stenosis, a severe narrowing of the larynx which made it difficult for him to breathe. The result was the need for a tracheostomy which required him to remain in the hospital for many weeks. As I got to know him and his family, I found it interesting to engage with him and learn his way of communicating at the time. Little did I know then that I would end up with baby communication being a focus towards the end of my career in neonates. James was one of the babies with sub-glottic stenosis resulting from the friction caused by the size of his endotracheal tube. As I look back now, it could have been prevented, however, when struggling to expand a baby's lungs with positive pressure ventilation, the endo-tracheal tube was considered a minor complication. I often wonder about James and his development over the years he would be 42 years old now! I am sure nurses think about the babies they have cared for; I have been challenged by memories of the babies who did not do so well and ended up with a life-long disability.

When you graduate with a qualification such as neonatal nursing, you were challenged by others who had grand expectations of your knowledge and how you would apply this to your caring. When I completed the 'JBCNS 400' neonatal course at University College Hospital in 1976, my course colleagues and I were enthusiastic as together we discovered the newly examined world of neonates. A fascination that held us in awe and being taught by the best was certainly a privilege. My course mate Cherry Bond is a leader today for her work on massage and infant engagement. Our paths have crossed several times over the years as we both developed a similar focus for newborn care. These contacts you make over the years provide a network of neonatal nurses who contribute to future collaborations and research opportunities.

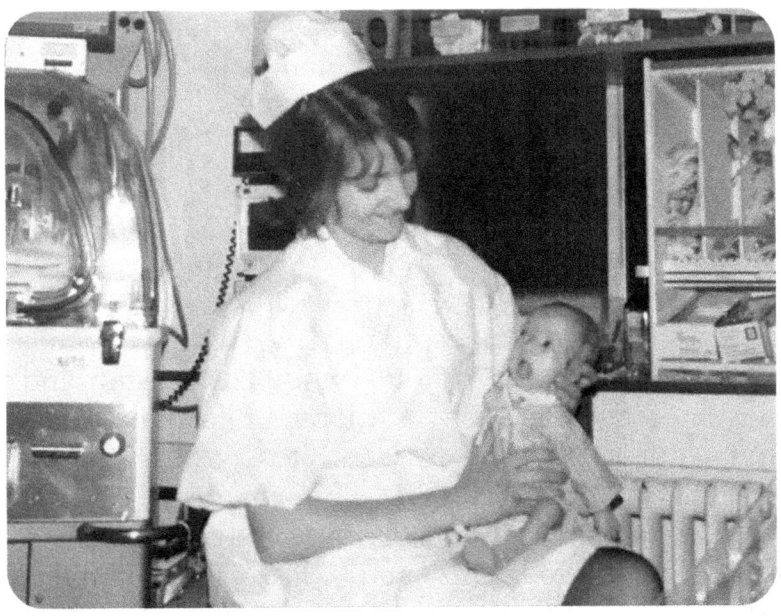

1976 – University College Hospital in London. Kaye learning about babies' communication.

I took a job at the London Hospital in the notorious east end. I was challenged by the low socio-economic groups of families whose babies we cared for, they were unique and mysterious to me. The mothers and babies came from many diverse cultural groups, and they taught me so much about relationships, hardship, and determination. This was good as I had the dual role of charge nurse as well as the educator and course coordinator. These joint roles would be unheard of today with so much specialisation and sub-specialisation. The three roles were challenging and exhausting but rewarding. I instructed groups of registered nurses, direct-entry midwives and enrolled nurses, all with different levels of understanding and critical inquiry. I found this challenge interesting, and it taught me that you can put a diverse group together if you take an individualised approach to teaching and learning. Sometimes I felt like I needed to pull my hair out with frustration as concepts went over the head of some and the impatience of others was very trying. I was proud of my job in neonatal nursing and the opportunities I had. One of my best achievements was having the neonatal course at the London Hospital accredited by the Joint Board of Clinical Studies (JBCNS), no easy feat. The JBCNS was an organisation instrumental in standardising the curricula for neonatal nursing courses across the UK and I believe added to the body of knowledge that enabled the profession to advance.

At the London Hospital my job sometimes required me to go on external transport in an ambulance to retrieve sick babies from other hospitals. I was obliged to change from the in-house uniform of a white cotton shift and put on the elaborate and very traditional uniform of a London Hospital nurse, we were expected to show a professional image. Pleated starched blue uniform dress, ragamuffin sleeves, large flat pearl buttons the size of a 50-cent piece, starched collars and cuffs, and a lace cap that had been pleated by a woman specifically employed for the job. I felt I was unique and special. I remember standing on a round-a-bout in outer London in this uniform with the infant in a crib with the ventilator which were mounted on an old English pram. I had an inexperienced female doctor with me who was terrified. The ambulance had broken down and we were standing next to the van waiting for another. We must have looked a sight and onlookers probably thought I was the nurse, the doctor the mother, and the baby a doll. Little did they know that this was a life-and-death situation. The replacement ambulance was an antiquated three-wheeled vehicle. I didn't feel too safe as it screeched around corners as the vehicle was very unstable. Thankfully, we all survived and arrived back in the neonatal intensive care unit in one piece. How times have changed. Now we have the highly technical expertise of the Newborn Emergency Transport Service (NETS) which has become a sub-specialty of neonatology. More about this in later essays.

Neonatal nursing: change and challenges

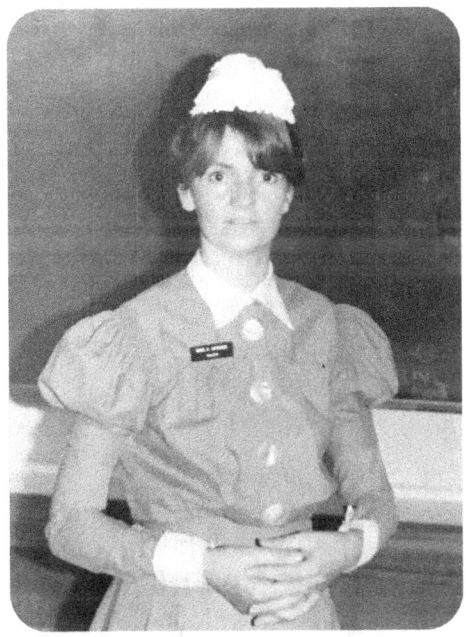

1979 - The London Hospital uniform, very traditional

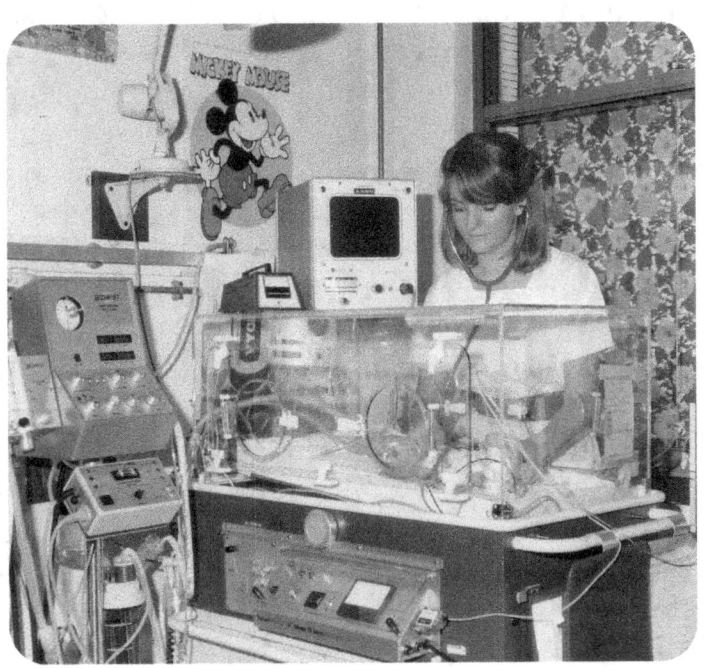

1980 – Kaye at The London Hospital, Whitechapel

When I worked the night shift, I was challenged by the allocation to care for four babies in one room with all four possibly on life support requiring mechanical ventilation. During a twelve-hour shift I had to have vigilance, expertise, knowledge, critical thinking, assertiveness, and multi-skilling. All traits contributed to my eventual leadership within neonatal nursing. When I hear nurses today say they are too busy to complete certain tasks I remember those days in London and just nod knowingly and smile. The 1970s the UK were in a state of crisis for newborn care and poor coverage by doctors meant tasks to keep the babies' condition stable fell to the nurses. We intubated, inserted the intravenous cannula, made feeding decisions, supported the parents, and triaged the admissions to the NICU. I balked at the intubation workshops that used kittens or stillborn infants as the mannequins. I thought this was barbaric. There was little support for nurses at this time and overtime was often demanded. You just did it. While it proved to be an excellent training field, I shudder at the memory of things we used to do. How did we survive, how did the babies survive?

While at the London Hospital I had the opportunity to meet Dr. Marshall Klaus, who was considered the father of neonatology, a pioneer in recognition of bonding relationships between mothers and their small sick babies. I had read his book (Maternal-Infant Bonding) and used it as a reference for my practice. He was visiting the neonatal unit at the invitation of Dr. Graeme Snodgrass, Head of the Department in 1979. I watched him talk with and support a young West Indian mother which was a lesson for me, and he encouraged the nurses to follow his lead. This image has remained firmly imprinted on my memory. When I think of neonatal nursing in 2022, the support and involvement of parents as partners with the nurses in caring for sick babies are the primary focus. I do wonder about all those families of babies born in the 1970s who struggled without this recognition. Marshall Klaus spoke of the nurses as "mothering the mothers," an expression I often use today. Now in 2022, we have younger nurses and older mothers, so maybe this saying takes on a different meaning with these groups. I think young nurses with little life experience must find it hard to support a new mother to hold and feed their babies. I have tried to support these nurses as it is paramount they still are in the specialty and eventually become part of the experienced team.

The profession of nursing has seen the rise of different specialties over the years. I had the privilege to be present at the London Hospital when the Neonatal Nurses Association (NNA) was first set up in the UK in 1978. This group achieved the goal to unite nurses across all hospitals as well as keep a level of standardisation for clinical practice. Informal gatherings of influential women took place, and the goals and rules were debated. Leaders such as Paula Hale, Anthea Blake, and Barbara Weller were involved. In the years to come these women influenced the development of neonatal nursing as a specialty in the UK and eventually in Australia. I was lucky to have known these powerful women over the years. As I think back to those times and the later professional organisations that emerged, I feel lucky to have been involved in the establishment of specialty organisations Australian Neonatal Nurses Association (ANNA) and the Council of International Neonatal Nurses (COINN), we have come a long way. Each of these women contributed to the specialty in their own unique way.

Meanwhile in Australia neonatal nursing started to emerge as a sub-specialty but it remained wedged between midwifery and paediatrics. A small specialty course for nurses working with neonates started in 1973 at John Spence Nursery, Royal Prince Alfred Hospital in Sydney. You had to be a midwife to do a neonatal course then - now we take in new graduates directly from university. The course started because of the increased demand for cots for premature newborns. This trend was also seen in other states across Australia and was kept with global trends. As the number of preterm births increased, the neonatal units were challenged to have trained nurses as there was an increase in the demand for cots which were predominately for preterm infants, we saw a trend of an extended length of hospital stay for weeks or months. I often thought of the effect on the families of being separated from their babies for so long, many were from the country and had to travel hours to spend a fleeting time with their babies.

When I returned to Australia in 1982, I was proud of the many clinical skills and knowledge I had acquired, and I felt I was ready to cement my career in the fledging specialty of neonatal nursing in Australia. I secured a position in Baxter Ward at the Royal Alexandra Hospital for Children in Sydney, a return to my alma mater. This was timely as the first neonatologist, Dr. George Williams, was appointed as Head of Neonatology. Until this time neonates were still seen as a part of paediatrics, and their care was managed by general paediatricians and anaesthetists. It was exciting to be part of this growing specialty in Australia. Over the decades nurses have had increased responsibility for the care of these vulnerable patients and their impact is evident in the educated nursing workforce of today.

One thing that was guaranteed through nursing was the opportunity to learn. The decades of the 80s and 90s saw an explosion of available information. Changes occurred across Australia, and these were often in isolation from developments in the different states that occurred in an ad hoc way. Nurses tended to work in silos of practice, even within their hospitals. This is still seen today in certain units. I sometimes thought this was a bad thing, but it was the one thing that eventually brought nurses together.

Baxter Ward at the Royal Alexandra Hospital for Children (RAHC) was the designated Neonatal Intensive Care Unit, with Grace Ward the specialty ward for surgical babies recovering from their operations who often had complex feeding needs. Each of the wards was managed by an amazing woman who had incredible nursing expertise; Shirley Watts and Chris Hynen. These expert and influential women were held in high esteem by doctors from all paediatric sub-specialties. I often reflect on their skills and what made them such leaders. It was their clinical ability and their no-nonsense approach to staff management attributes that can be seen in few of the managers today. I have worked with many nurse managers since and some have become good friends. I believe the role of clinical nurse consultant and nurse manager are complementary to each other and some of the best experiences I had was working with Jenny Elliott. We had mutual respect and although Jenny was often seen as formidable, she had a soft heart and really cared about the team. Recognition of these pioneers of neonatal nursing has dwindled as history and its contribution to current practice receives little acknowledgment. I am dismayed at this as history can teach us so much. I often say if you stand still long enough the same issues and problems present, this cycle is about seven years in my estimate. If you pay attention, it can prevent the same mistakes from being made.

I arrived in this environment fired up from the recognition and expertise I had gained in my leadership role in neonatal nursing in London. I was a manager, an educator, and a skilled clinical nurse. However, I was quickly put in my place by the antiquated nursing culture and the powerful establishment of the current rank and file RAHC nurses. Most had not worked in another hospital and believed the time worked in a particular unit for months or years equated to knowledge and expertise in neonatal nursing gained across other hospitals. This was typical of nursing in this era, there was no recognition of prior learning in another NICU. So, despite a glowing reference and years at the highest level, I was relegated to the lowest rung on the ladder. My learning had begun! The year was 1982.

The NICU at RAHC was crowded with small babies, the majority were on life support. The equipment was clumsy and primitive by today's standards. As nurses, we learned how to troubleshoot the antiquated Campbell ventilators by removing the bellows and looking for splits that had occurred in the rubber, the inspiratory to expiratory ratios were guesswork on what sounded right to the person setting them. We were taught to breathe with the machine to decide if the settings were right. Contrasting this to the sophisticated computerised machines we have today is a little like comparing the Wright Brothers' Flying machines to the A380. Certain practices now rely on technology and an underlying understanding of the basic principles may be missing.

The care practices were based on what was considered as best practice of the time. The mechanical ventilation was harsh on small delicate lungs and air leaks (pneumothoraces) were plentiful as the air under pressure leaked into the surrounding tissue. Sounds horrific. Surfactant was just beginning to be used in clinical practice to reduce the compliance of the small stiff lungs. It was not unusual for one baby to have up to six chest drains to expand their small stiff noncompliant lungs. This was a challenge for nurses who had to expertly change the tubing and keep the drains working and bubbling 24 hours a day, so the baby's lungs did not collapse. A skill lost today with the use of surfactant and less invasive therapies being customary practice. Intravenous feeding was slowly being used more often, along with the associated complications of extravasation, lipidaemia, and cholestatic jaundice. The rate of these complications has diminished over time. Do we become more proficient or are we more vigilant? We learned from these complications and refined our clinical and diagnostic skills. Negotiating the challenges of the past have enabled us to give safe and effective care today. History is an important teacher, and it needs to be part of the curricula of current neonatal courses.

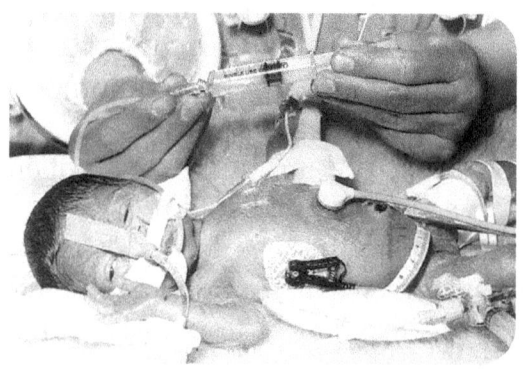

1983 – Newborn care in the early days

Neonatal Surgery had become routine with smaller and sicker infants needing a surgical intervention. Surgeons were cautious and anaesthetists had control of post-operative care, including ventilation and pain relief. With the employment of two neonatologists, Dr. George Williams and Dr. Andrew Berry, the post-operative care shifted to these specialists. Nurses had gained expertise in caring for neonates in the post-operative period and eventually, the recovery ward was bypassed as the babies were transferred directly from the operating theatre back to the NICU. This was in recognition of the skills of both neonatal doctors and nurses, and these trends were simultaneously occurring in other NICUs across all states of Australia. However, there was little interaction between the nurses in the units across Australia and practices varied according to individual preferences and policies. That started to change as nurses and doctors attended the same conferences, namely the Australian Perinatal Society (APS) which became the Perinatal Society of Australia and new Zealand (PSANZ)

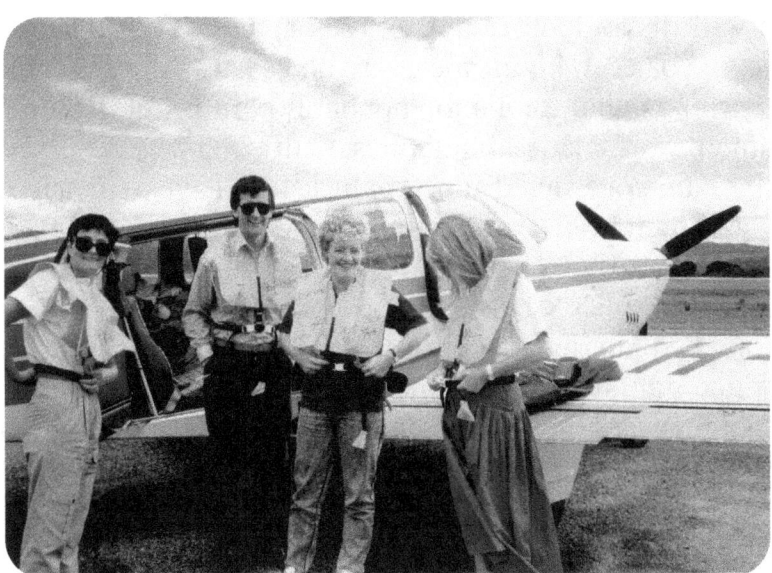

1987 – On our way to the perinatal conference (PSANZ) in Launceston. Pilot Andrew Berry, Victoria Cullens, Janette Tommasi, and Kaye. Life jackets were needed as we flew across the Bass Straight from mainland Australia to Tasmania.

A baby's pain was managed by the anaesthetists and adequate pain management was identified as a concern for nurses who had to try to comfort babies who were in pain. Linda Johnston (now Dean at the University of Toronto) and I undertook a survey of attitudes to pain management for post-operative care in neonates. We needed to show the differences if we were to improve pain management. This was our first foray into research, and it was 1984. Although this was a rocky start to research, we received criticism about our questionnaire, we did however manage to provoke a discussion about newborn pain that has continued for years. Today pain is one of the most emotive topics in the NICU and nurses continually name it as a topic for research in their university assignments. When pain assessment tools were introduced, the discussion became more objective and the management of pain in the NICU for post-operative infants improved, as infants were able to be comfortable and relatively pain-free. In a conversation years later with Dr. Neil Campbell from Royal Children's Hospital in Melbourne, Victoria, he challenged me about pain assessment strategies and commented that "neonatal pain will drive doctors and nurses apart". That discussion has come back to haunt me over the years as nurses took on the baton as champions for neonatal pain relief. Recently a comment was made about nurses altering the pain scores so the babies received more pain relief. I was surprised at this comment as it undermines the integrity of nurses' observations, the debate continues. Small premature infants in perinatal units struggled and suffered through intensive care as the pain debate continued. The national PEGS (pain evidence gap study) was one of the first attempts to gain consistency across 24 NICUs in Australia. Luckily today pain assessment and management is a fundamental practice and all clinicians work together to alleviate suffering. This has been a relief for me as I did often wonder if the message would ever be heard.

Collaboration with doctors and how they perceived nurses and nursing practice has been an interesting dynamic over the past decades. The hierarchical paternalistic system gradually gave way to a more peer partnership model. This was mostly built around relationships and personality. I had many friendly but firm discussions with one of our old school neonatologists (Dr. Bruce Story) on the role of nurses and their quest for higher degrees, I saw red when he insisted on calling us 'sisters'. This unresolved debate he took to his grave. Typically nurses and doctors worked together in the NICU where teamwork was a priority, and respect for each other developed. I remember when I started work back in Baxter Ward, I worked with a new senior registrar who became our fellow (now Professor Paul Colditz). He was new to the NICU, I was new to the unit, and we worked together building on each other's knowledge and trust. Both of us admitted we were flying blind in terms of policy and practice guidelines. It was a good example of teamwork. I could name many examples of good teamwork where the babies' outcomes were improved by working together. We still work together in diverse ways in different units and different states - a testament to the power of relationships and networks we build throughout our careers.

The 1980s proved a challenge in clinical care. I look at some of the images of babies that I have collected from that time, and I cringe at the practices of the time. At one stage, sheepskins were considered the newest strategy to help with pressure points and skincare. However, looking back at photographs you can see a baby lying prone on their abdomen, head twisted to one side, arms at awkward angles due to large cumbersome boards securing intravenous cannula that restricted movement, legs extended with hips adducted. It looks like torture. When I compare this image to one of today with a baby nicely flexed, side-lying, head in midline and arms forward with hands available for self-consolation on their face, I find myself in an 'ah' moment of satisfaction.

Throughout the two decades of the 80s and 90s substantial changes occurred in neonatal services across Australia as hospitals merged and new intensive care units were set up. There were nursing shortages in all states and in the early 90s the NSW Government recruited experienced neonatal nurses from the UK and Ireland to fill these shortages. The acuity and numbers of babies in the NICUs were growing due to the increased survival rates of low birth-weight infants and, when new intensive care units were set up, the nurse shortage increased. The recruitment of international nurses was not supported by the nurses' unions and picket lines were formed in front of hospitals that employed these 'scab' nurses. Interestingly, many of these nurses remained and have become an essential part of the stable and experienced workforce of today.

In 1989 a report into Maternity Services, which included Neonatal Services was commissioned in NSW and chaired by Professor Rodney Shearman, a respected obstetrician. It became known as the Shearman Report and was instrumental in setting the standard for neonatal services, many of which remain today. The recommendations from the report saw the recognition of the value of nursing through recommended nurse-to-patient ratios, however, the implementation was unsuccessful. This is still a regret of mine, as we continue to campaign for ratios and safe staffing numbers today. The report did recommend the establishment of post-discharge home visiting services with teams of experienced nurses funded to enable babies to be discharged home earlier, thereby freeing up beds in the NICU. These services allowed nurses to expand into new roles and different contexts. Some of these services stay in a few hospitals and others have seen the funding amalgamated into general NICU services.

I had the honour, together with Heather Mann a Clinical Nurse Consultant from Newcastle in New South Wales, when we were the neonatal nurse representative on the NSW Health Department neonatal working group with the brief to review neonatal services and make recommendations for future planning. These were interesting times as we struggled to make our voices heard in the competing needs of neonatologists to direct the recommendations to improve neonatal services. We were successful in getting recognition for the education of nurses and clinical nurse educators were employed in each NICU. Our various visits to NICUs and SCNs across the state enabled us to name frontline issues, mostly associated with shortages and specialty training. I am sure if I repeated those visits today the same issues would be mentioned. This shows that often solutions are short term and a longer vision for strategic planning needs to have more nursing involvement for sustainment.

Out of these recommendations, the Perinatal Services Network (PSN) was set up with Professor David Henderson-Smart (DHS) as the Director in the early 90s. I now see this was the biggest change for neonatal services and the subsequent care provided. DHS, as he was affectionately known, was supportive of nurses and saw their value, not only in expert clinical care but in the standardisation of practices and benchmarking practices across different hospitals to improve patient outcomes. Under his influence nurses became part of working groups of managers, educators and consultants, and the sharing of information, resources and ideas led to better practices. The collection of audit data by experienced neonatal nurses across Australia enabled outcomes of various practices to be shown and units with good outcomes were placed as a gold standard for benchmarking. Outcomes were identified such as Intraventricular Haemorrhage (IVH), chronic lung disease (CLD), retinopathy of prematurity (ROP), infection, use of parenteral nutrition, and growth. Follow-up clinics enabled developmental outcomes to be measured and became routine in most hospitals across Australia. You could say that neonatal services across Australia were at their best.

I have wandered down memory lane and as memories appeared, I wrote. However, with all these advancements neonatal nurses continued to struggle with high acuity, inadequate staff numbers, and a lack of support for continuing education. Education was a cornerstone of nursing practice and recognition came with the combination of resources when courses were amalgamated across hospitals. In my following essays, you will see how these changes had an impact on the professional standing of neonatal nurses as well as advancements in clinical practice and eventually neonatal nursing becoming a specialty.

Essay Three

Early Days of Learning

When you start on your journey to becoming a nurse you also start a journey of learning. Nursing and the many teachers I have had taught me so much and left an impression on me that I often take into my teaching. Learning is lifelong and even today after over 40 years of nursing I am still learning.

In 1988 I undertook a course - A Diploma in Teaching at Sydney College of Advanced Education, later this college was incorporated into the University of Sydney. This was to become part of my learning as I had been appointed as the Nurse Educator in the NICU. I was excited to be appointed to this position, however there was a lot of resistance from the 'old guard' as I call them. Maybe it was professional jealousy and the lack of recognition of my previous experiences which included being a nurse educator when I was in London. I felt a qualification was necessary to enable me to advance in my education career. My classes were held early evening and my classmates from all areas of nursing are still friends and acquaintances today, a common bond you might say. It was interesting being on the other side of teaching as part of the assessment of the course was for a tutor to sit in a class and observe me as I taught a lesson. I wasn't too enthralled by the idea. The allocated teacher/assessor whose name was Shirley came to my session on neonatal jaundice, a topic I did not particularly like. Shirley had the reputation of being a 'hard' examiner. Also, in the class sitting in the back was Peter Barr who had recently joined our team in Baxter as a neonatologist. Peter said he was keen to see how nurses were being taught! This experience taught me that I needed to get used to having challenging people in my audience. I remember Peter coming up to me after the class saying "Kaye, my notes fit on a postage stamp." I have always remembered that and to this day try to speak in presentations without notes. Shirley's feedback was "well that was a dud." Despite this, she gave me a good grade – never underestimate an assessor. When I was an assessor for nursing students at RAHC I remember failing several in their clinical skills assessments. This was met with different responses. I might add that two nurses went on to become nursing leaders. Maybe failure or poor feedback triggers you to do better.

I did go on and convert my diploma to a Bachelor of Education in Nursing making to drive each term to Armidale with a colleague and friend for the residentials. We shared a room and laughed about the class divisions that occurred between educators and managers during the common subjects. I recall the managers were such an unruly lot, so disruptive, yet today they are the most senior nurses in the state. Armed with the knowledge and experience I gained in education and teaching I was ready for the challenges that awaited me.

Neonatal nursing became a specialty as it developed its own unique body of knowledge. The course at Royal Prince Alfred Hospital (RPAH) was well established and the team at RAHC was approached to join for a combined course. In the past the RPAH students came to RAHC for their clinical experience with babies who required surgery. Many of them stayed and became part of our specialist workforce. Combining with RPAH was to become a steppingstone for future collaborations that ultimately strengthened the profession. Jean Naylor was the course coordinator, and I became her sidekick, often challenging assumptions. I became colleagues with other leaders in the specialty and my collaboration and friendship with Sandie Bredemeyer, the Clinical Nurse Educator at RPAH, resulted in a new direction for neonatal nursing and a lifelong friend. Sandie was a leader as she was inspirational with recognition for her knowledge and vision for clinical nursing.

Also, at this time the undergraduate education for nursing moved from a hospital-based certificate into the Higher Education Sector with various universities starting degree programs. There was considerable opposition from the nursing establishment with criticism focused on the seemingly unprepared graduate nurses as they entered the workforce. I didn't hold this view as so many motivated and skilled nurses joined the nursing workforce. You could say they enriched nursing and certainly added to the knowledge and expansion of nursing roles. I remember our first new graduate to be employed in Baxter NICU, Renee Mountenay (Muirhead), who defied all odds and showed her potential and is now a clinical nurse consultant undertaking her PhD in Brisbane, Queensland. Students undertook clinical placements on rotation which gave them some idea of the different contexts within nursing and the health sector. The responsibility for education for nurses wanting to specialise fell to the individual hospitals. Therefore, the neonatal nursing courses which were expanding became vital for the development and indeed the survival of the specialty of neonatal nursing.

The combined courses of Royal Prince Alfred Hospital and RAHC expanded further with the collaboration of three other tertiary hospitals in Sydney, Royal North Shore Hospital, Prince of Wales Children's Hospital, and Royal Hospital for Women. Bringing together students from the five hospitals ultimately brought together nurses from these hospitals and then more as we started to become a specialty within New South Wales. We started to see graduate nurses enter these neonatal nursing programs and they brought with them skills in critical thinking and evidence-based practice. I welcomed these nurses as if it was the beginning of the future – at least that was how I saw it.

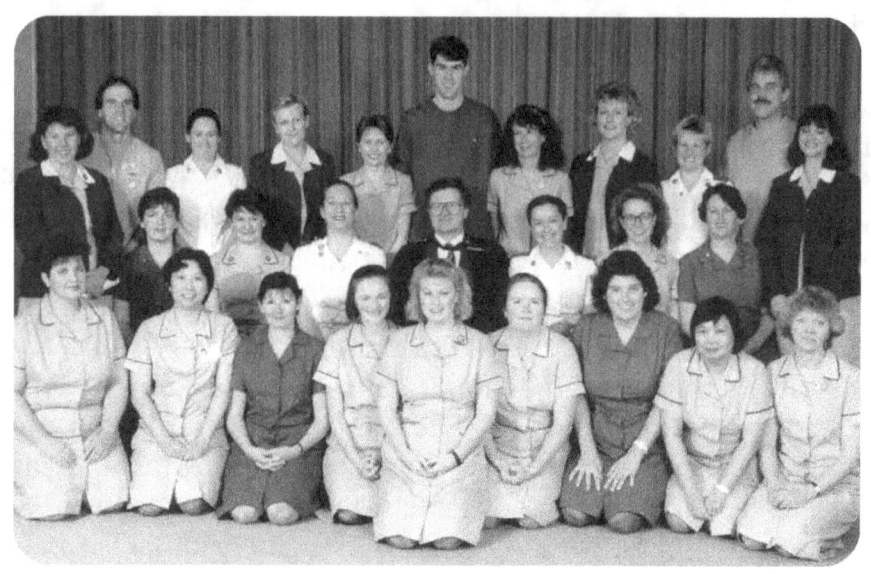

1989. The first combined neonatal course with students from Royal Alexandra Hospital for Children, Royal Prince Alfred Hospital, Royal North Shore Hospital, Royal Hospital for Women and Prince of Wales Children's Hospital. Health Minister Hon Peter Collins partly funded the course.

As the courses developed and expanded so too did clinical practice. With the expansion of technology, nurses were being challenged to become technicians as well as carers. There was a risk that nurses were giving away the caring components of their role as the technology became more sophisticated and, in some cases more interesting. In addition, technology was opening clinical as well as ethical challenges. When I look back on the skills we gained from learning the equipment, troubleshooting failures and seeking innovative practices, I see nurses as the conductor of the intensive care environment. So often we had to fix tubes and leads and at the same time ensure the safety of the small person we were caring for. To this day I believe nurses make the best plumbers for finding solutions, a skill I found handy on several occasions in my home.

Clinical nurses contributed to the expansion of knowledge and many practices developed from a trial-and-error scenario. Skincare was a concern and we saw terrible abrasions and scarring from the overzealous use of electrodes, tapes, and equipment. I saw nurses create innovative taping practices to secure tubes, cut to size equipment to be suitable for the smallest baby, use sheepskins to avoid pressure points, and liberally use Eucren when it was first available. Managing to catch a slippery baby in your hands was a skill in itself. Nurses learned from doing and gained knowledge as they went about their daily routines. Teaching occurred at the cot-side when novice nurses partnered with more experienced nurses. This remains one of the best and most wanted ways of teaching today. Working with an experienced role model has a dual role, the learner learns from the best, and the teacher has the satisfaction that they have imparted their knowledge.

With the expansion of the specialty of neonatal nursing, we started to see changes in the way nurses were taught. I remember when I did my course in London most of the content was taught by doctors. This continued in Australia, but we began to see more nurses take on some of the traditional doctor topics. Nurses started to present at seminars and conferences held in small hospitals throughout the state. The first seminar I spoke at was at Katoomba in the Blue Mountains west of Sydney. It was a Paediatric Nurses Outreach Seminar. This was memorable for several reasons. I was asked to speak on two topics, Transporting Neonates, and Jaundice – the dreaded Jaundice will forever haunt me! In the audience in the front row was the Director of Nursing and in the back of the room was my husband. I was nervous on both counts especially when a 'Professor of Indian descent' spoke on resuscitation and mentioned that in some primitive countries, like Cyprus, they used the beak of a pelican to stimulate a baby to breathe. I was terrified that my husband, who grew up in Cyprus, would call out. Some things are unpredictable, and I will always remember these presentations and how nervous I was. I did survive and have gone on to present at many conferences, local, national, and international levels. I relish the opportunity to present, and I find I look for innovative ways to get the message across. I must say that as we move into virtual teaching, I believe there are only so many hours of ZOOM one can take! You can't beat that interaction you get from a live audience.

When I think about events that were significant when neonatal nursing moved into the Higher Education Sector, four come to mind. As part of the initiative of the NSW Government to recruit and retain nurses in the specialty of neonatal nursing, they funded a Neonatal Course at the NSW College of Nursing. This was to replace the hospital courses which were subjected to intermittent funding and cancellations. Positions were secured in this course for nurses from each of the nine NICUs in Sydney and Newcastle. A positive outcome was the friendships and collegiality that formed across all NICUs. After about five years, this course also became a victim of funding cuts and many universities sought to attract the popular specialty to their programs. There was competition from universities, and I am not sure if this was the best outcome for the specialty. Universities have an agenda and they do not necessarily meet the requirements of the clinical specialty and may cancel or reschedule courses to their convenience.

The University of Western Sydney took the initiative and started a Graduate Diploma in Neonatal Nursing at the MacArthur Campus in Campbelltown. Despite being such a long way away this course resulted in two notable events for neonatal nursing as I see it. The first was the Head of School, Margaret McMillan, who was one of the most inspirational nurse leaders of the time and for the next several decades. She had a vision that I found enlightening for nurses and nursing to lead the way in health care. She challenged us to re-think traditional curricular and teaching styles and turn the focus on the students being responsible for their own learning. The second event was a research study undertaken using four of the students in the course. I was excited to be involved in this study as I was learning from an expert, Professor Jenny Greenwood, who had a wicked sense of humour. She taught me about a new methodology for gathering information from clinical nurses. It was called 'think aloud' and the nurses wore microphones and recorders and just spoke about what they were doing as they did their clinical caregiving. What a revelation as I entered the thoughts of the nurses 'time for midday cares, temperature, mouth care, nappy change' those words have sung loudly for years. Each time I have met up with Jenny over the years she uses these words as a type of slogan for neonatal nursing. All these tapes were transcribed and then coded. I got to know Jann Foster, a neonatal nurse who was working as a research assistant to Jenny. The days spent coding the transcripts were such a hoot as Jann and I agreed we were neonatal nurses and we had to convince the academic of what the expressions and terminology meant. I think this is where I became aware of how neonatal nurses talk in 'jargon speak'. Some very lively discussions took place. The resulting publications are still used as a window into neonatal nursing, how nurses think, and how they are socialised into the NICU.

Neonatal nurses slowly began to participate in research and these early roles were often as followers of protocols set by doctors. Over time, this started to change and, I believe as nurses gained more critical thinking skills they challenged practices and started to ask questions such as why? My early exploration of research was to jump in at the top end with a randomised controlled trial of using a suction adaptor for suctioning a baby's ETT. When I found my ethics application in a file at home, I gasped as it was handwritten, and the lack of detail was embarrassing by today's standards. Still, someone must have seen some potential in me as it was approved with a small grant to enable it to start. It was 1986 and I employed my first research assistant, what an achievement and it made me feel so important.

My first research assistant was Linda Johnston, and you have heard about her progress. She went on to obtain a PhD working in the laboratory with white mice. For those who know Linda, this was typical of her quest for hard science that she wanted to give back to nursing to improve our scientific basis. Other early nurse researchers who made a huge contribution to the knowledge base for neonatal nursing were Jane Davey, Sandie Bredemeyer, Carmel Collins, and Jann Foster who led the way for neonatal nurses to undertake PhDs. Today we have seen a proliferation of neonatal nurses doing PhDs and the profession and specialty has become richer for this trend as they set critical inquiry into the curricula for all education programs.

Linda Johnston went on to become the first Professor of Neonatal Nursing in Australia. This was of such significance and took the specialty to the next step on the proverbial ladder of recognition. The University of Melbourne showed great insight with this appointment, and we saw neonatal nurses starting to influence the direction of clinical practice, education, and research.

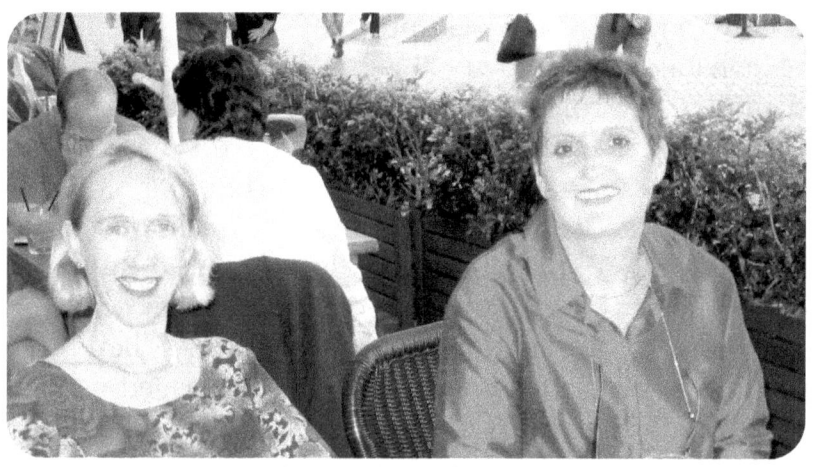

Linda Johnston (right) and Denise Harrison – two influential nurses for neonatal research.

Education and research influenced clinical practice and we saw the development and implementation of competencies. Jan Andrews from the NSW College of Nursing worked with us in identifying the specific components of clinical practice where safety was a concern and nurses needed to be competent in their practice. These standards gave the specialty a framework to define our practice. The next step was the development of specific neonatal nursing competencies, and the standards were originally developed by the Clinical Nurse Consultant group under the leadership of Sandie Bredemeyer. The baton was handed over to Maureen West who continued to update the competency standards with a team of expert clinical neonatal nurses. Looking back to those times, I don't think we understood the impact of our work on the practices today.

I remember nurses from many different hospitals working in groups sharing their experiences and driving the specialty forward. I see their influence today and I will acknowledge them in another essay.

Essay Four

Transporting babies: on the road to advanced practice

Neonatal services had become regionalized out of necessity. With the vast nature of Australia, it was a challenge to ensure all babies born in any hospital could be transferred to the level of service they needed. In the 1980s there were around 200 hospitals in NSW. These ranged from small cottage hospitals in small rural communities to the larger tertiary hospitals in the cities. Equity of access for all babies born meant that a mobile unit had to bring them to the city.

In 1982 when I first started in Baxter Ward at RAHC, I worked with two people who were to become instrumental in the establishment of Newborn Transport Services in NSW. The first was Andrew Berry, a new neonatologist with a passion not only for transporting newborn babies across the state but also for ensuring they were stabilised for the move. He recognised the inherent danger in caring for babies in mobile environments and the necessity of having skilled professionals to do this. The second person to mention was Julie McNall who was to lead a team of transport nurses who took on these advanced practice roles. When I first met Julie at orientation in 1982, I am sure this was not on her radar, her focus was on the immediate caring needs of newborn babies in intensive care.

When I was in London, I had taken part in transporting babies from two different hospitals with very different approaches. One story I have already told you (waiting on a round-a-bout) and there are many more. There were no teams and nurses, and doctors were plucked from the clinical areas as the need arose to retrieve a sick baby. The equipment was innovative, and you prayed that it would not fail. It was a potluck who your team was and sometimes you prayed that certain doctors were not on duty. I remember being in the ambulance with one doctor who sucked on the alcohol mediwipes for the whole journey, "to calm my nerves" he said. Well, imagine the confidence I didn't have with him. There were no sophisticated communication lines or mobile phones, so messages were often relayed from a landline to the doctor trying to intubate a very small baby. Often it was their first time, and it was scary.

The London Hospital was in the east end of London and most of the retrieval came from a sister hospital about 3 km up the road, traffic was so congested, that retrievals could take ages. Again, we were called away from our clinical duties. We wore hospital scrubs in the clinical area, however, when you were called out for retrieval you had to change into your full traditional London hospital uniform. The collars and cuffs had to be folded and placed around your neck and wrists. This took a huge amount of time so in the interest of having to move quickly to catch the ambulance, I stitched mine to my uniform. It worked a treat until one day the Matron entered the lift, she took hold of my wrist, ran her finger around my neck, and told me "London nurses wear their uniforms correctly". I felt as though I could sit on a six-pence. Uniforms have always had a role in transport. I remember when the team was set up in Sydney, Julie, the nurse consultant, wanted the nurses to wear culottes, a challenge for the conservative establishment. Julie eventually won; however, her designer model was not supported! Today looking at the NETS (Newborn Emergency Transport Service) nurses they are kitted out in emergency overalls with fluoro bands around their legs; a far cry from the regimented nursing uniforms meant to be worn with pride.

Working in the mobile environment of intensive care was a challenge and required critical thinking skills and decisions made on the run. Many nurses were not suited to this type of nursing, or it took them a while to adjust. Clinical expertise was essential as you never knew what the unexpected held. When retrieval was first started in Baxter Ward in 1983 or thereabouts, there was a lot of excitement. The vigilance of Andrew Berry as well as his skills, attention to detail, and ability to describe over the phone how to solve just about any problem with the equipment made him ideal for setting up the service. I remember his wife telling me that she could troubleshoot the old ventilator circuits and their temperamental valves as she had heard Andrew describe the solution so often in the middle of the night.

Andrew was a good teacher and, although at times you thought he was not listening, or watching, nothing escaped him. One day I was asked to do a retrieval from Mona Vale Hospital on Sydney's northern beaches as all other available staff were on existing retrievals. So off I went with Andrew. I remember commenting to him that it was a nuisance as I had just had my nails painted for a special function that evening. You know he made me hand-ventilate the baby back and those old Ambu bags were difficult to use, especially when you're trying to keep your nails pristine! I caught him with a smirk on his face, he knew exactly what he wanted to do, cheeky. That was probably the end of my transport days; I left it to the emerging team of experts.

In 1989 the NETS team was set up with dedicated nurses. Nurses were recruited to join the two Children's Hospitals in Sydney; they were experienced clinical nurses from many neonatal intensive care units across Sydney. Julie McNall was appointed as the Charge Nurse and was responsible for recruitment and training as well as providing input into the running of the service. This was certainly a time for nurses to prove themselves in this exciting and expanding role. I often thought this role was ideal for the development of the nurse practitioner as had occurred internationally. However, we still wait today for this advanced practice role to take a hold of the retrieval nurses. I did wonder if I would see this occur, hot off the press – an advertisement appeared this week in July. Other teams such as the retrieval team in Townsville, Queensland, had led the way with this role.

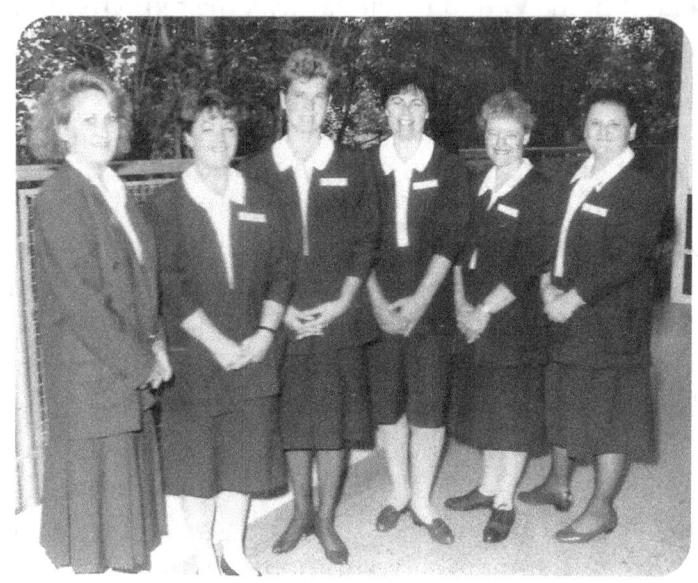

The NETS team at RAHC in 1989 – note the original culottes.

The nurses undertaking retrieval have advanced the specialty through their expert clinical skills and ability to lead and work within a multi-disciplinary team. I sometimes ponder on what makes a retrieval nurse. They must have vigilance as well as the ability to be insightful and empathetic as they gently tread into foreign territories of the NICU. Taking over the care and management of a baby where the nurses and doctors have spent many long hours caring, nurturing, and often resuscitating fragile neonates requires a special skill. The confidence the staff have in these nurses is complimentary and I believe often not acknowledged.

The Newborn retrieval service has grown exponentially over the past three decades. I feel so proud of this achievement as I watched and nurtured its growth over the years.

The legacy of those nurses who through their passion made the retrieval system work is strong. Many have moved on and when I look at the current NETS team of nurses familiar faces are few and far between. I asked my friend and colleague Julie McNall for a few words of reflection on her time setting up NETS. Here is what she had to say;

> *Looking back, it is difficult to identify any one aspect as it was all new, but my primary focus was to set up the nursing branch of the newborn transport system. It was important to have a solid foundation, and an excellent nursing reputation and be recognised as contributing to the improved survival and outcome of our sickest babies.*

One thing that we were often faced with as nurses was dealing with the unexpected. Retrieval nurses have had to deal with this a lot and Julie describes an incident that shows how you can never guess the outcome and sometimes it is luck that helps you out.

> *A memorable event occurred in December 1989 with the devastating earthquake in Newcastle. I returned to the ward around 10 am after another all-nighter on transport. As I crossed the road at the side of The Children's Hospital in Camperdown, there were a lot of trees. I remember there were no bird sounds. Animals know when something is coming. When I arrived at the NETS Office, I was told that an earthquake had hit Newcastle and they might need to move the babies from Newcastle. Andrew Berry and I quickly took off in the helicopter. The day ended around 10 pm following the transfer of a mother in premature labor, luck was on our side as we decided to take a midwife with us. Almost as soon as we took off all too soon a 32-week gestation baby arrived. Thankfully, the midwife was able to squeeze into the rear end of the helicopter (it was a rear load) to deliver the baby and I looked after the top end and baby: all ended well. I think the pilot on opening the door at the back never saw a women's birthing position in the same way again. When I arrived home that night, I was*

told I smelt strongly of petrol so maybe that's how we got through so many long hours - sniffing petrol.

The JKB Annual Seminar was set up in memory of Jo Kent Biggs who joined the service after six months and later became the Nurse Manager when Julie left. Tragically Jo died suddenly in 2016. The seminar was set up in her honour and has provided a platform for nurses to present their work, network with other retrieval nurses from across Australia, and highlight many developments in retrieval. The inaugural seminar was memorable as it brought together nurses who had worked together in those early days of retrieval.

When I reflect on the NETS Service, I am proud of how it has grown from a fledgling service of improvision to one of a team of highly skilled clinicians who take on many challenges as they integrate intensive care into a truly mobile service. In recent years the NETS service was moved away from a clinical hospital setting to Bankstown Aerodrome. I am saddened by this move as the NETS nurses have a lot to contribute by being an integrated service and it also affords the NETS team the opportunity to be at the cutting edge of nursing developments. Perhaps one day it will be reunited back into a clinical service. However, unless we have politicians who truly understand newborn care and the needs of those providing the service, I feel it is destined to remain separated for a long time.

I would like to see Nurse Practitioners lead the NETS Retrieval teams as this is where I believe nursing, especially neonatal nursing can shine. I hope sick and vulnerable newborn infants, whether preterm or term will be cared for by neonatal nurses. Neonates are a very different specialty group to Paediatrics.

Essay Five

Pioneers of neonatal nursing

Pioneers are those who forge the way for others to follow. When I think of pioneers I tend to think of covered wagons and a long trek into the unknown. Neonatal nursing was like that in the beginning. Some saw the vision and knew where we needed to head, others followed and took the journey further and then there were the laggards or sceptics who never thought we would make it. I want to dig into my memory and bring out the particular assets of those who I see as pioneers of neonatal nursing. There are numerous ways to be a pioneer and often it is the contribution of many that make the powerful surge forward.

Australia has its pioneers, but I will also refer to some of my international colleagues and friends who inspired me in my quest to lead the way in Australia. I am honoured to have known these women and men who have all left a little of themselves in me the way I hope I can leave a little of me in future and emerging leaders.

I first became aware of Judy Jamieson in the mid-eighties at several meetings of the Australian Perinatal Society (APS) as it was known then. This multidisciplinary society eventually became PSANZ (Perinatal Society of Australia and New Zealand). Judy was one of those nurses who had a presence and people tended to listen to what she said. I saw her as influential in the direction of specialist education for nurses and her influence on the transport nurses. She came from Melbourne (not that that mattered) but it did give her that aura of distance. Over the years we got to know each other more and had mutual respect. She influenced the way I thought about education and training, but it was her pedantic attention to detail that has stayed with me. Is this a positive trait to have?

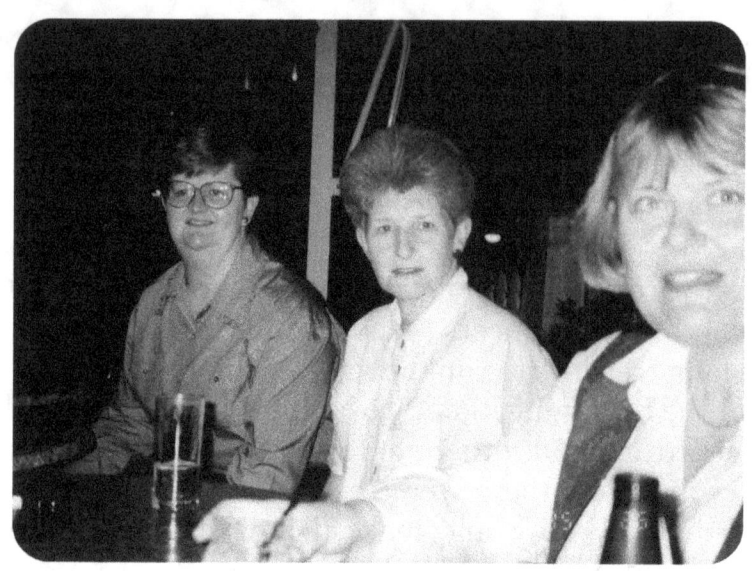

Judy Jamieson (Vic), Clare Doherty (Qld) and Sandie Bredemeyer (NSW) – pioneers in neonatal nursing

Peggy Taylor was often at meetings with Judy as she too came from Melbourne. I wonder what it was about Melbourne that produced these influencers? Peggy left an impression on me and neonatal nursing for three reasons; She was the first nurse I heard speak at a multi-disciplinary meeting about the nursing workforce, again in the mid-eighties. Before then it was unheard of, and the nursing workforce was not considered in the drive to expand neonatal services nationally. She campaigned for not only more nurses but specifically neonatal-trained nurses. Peggy became the first nurse to be President of PSANZ and she also received an AM. I followed in her footsteps as I became the second nurse to be PSANZ President and receive an AM. Two achievements of which I am immensely proud. Sadly, Peggy died in 2021 with little recognition from the neonatal nursing community. That got me thinking about why our legacies are not celebrated. Our history is so important for nurses to know and I want to make sure other pioneer nurses are remembered. One way is to celebrate them in this series of essays so newer neonatal nurses know of their achievements.

As we became more vocal in our quest to make neonatal nurses heard I am reminded of Jessie Everson who was cautious about moving too soon. Sometimes caution can be a barrier and being a risk taker can forge our paths. I was fired up with enthusiasm that the neonatal nurses of NSW needed to form a professional group. Jessie eventually became the first President of ANN – NSW (Association of Neonatal Nurses of NSW), I served as her honorary secretary. Jessie's caution annoyed me at the beginning, but I learned to listen and learn as she helped provide the foundation for the future of ANN. Sadly her legacy has also been forgotten.

At the same time, I got to know Sandie Bredemeyer who I believe is one of the truly inspiring pioneers of neonatal nursing in Australia. Sandie has an amazing intellect and her ability to critically work through some of those early struggles with calmness and humour was impressive. I saw us as partners as we saw things the same way and it was always good to bounce ideas off each other. Sandie became one of the first neonatal nurses in Australia to undertake a PhD and forged the path for others to follow. She was fair in her approach and she had the vision to ensure the specialty had the evidence to support the practice. We enjoyed each other's company and became good friends. Sandie was recognised by her peers and received an OAM for her services to neonatal nursing. She deserved this honour, and I am proud to have worked with her over many years.

It was through ANNA (Australian Neonatal Nurses Association) that I met Vicki Carson. Vicki was from Townsville in Queensland and had a fresh approach and a drive to make ANNA a success. She was a genuinely nice person and had an engaging smile and laugh, even in difficult circumstances. Vicki was a manager and showed the insight needed to make an organisation workable. She knew so much about organisations, governance, and finances, I felt ignorance in her presence. I have continued to draw on her ability for various consultations. She is passionate about nursing and that is a necessary trait for a pioneer.

There were so many other pioneers in their ways, and I acknowledge them silently. If I tried to mention them all I would fail and probably offend others by omission. However, I want to mention three who had a significant impact on me and my career and direction in neonatal nursing.

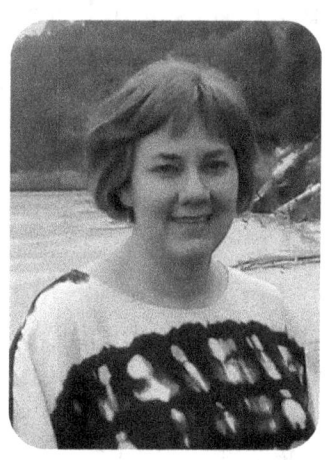

Vicki Carson at ACNN Conference on Fraser Island 2016.

The first is Linda Johnston who is a dear friend today. I first met Linda in Baxter Ward at The Royal Alexandra Hospital for Children, Sydney when she was recruited in the mid-eighties for her experience with neonates, having obtained her RN in the USA. This 'American' nurse as she was called, was both terrifying and admired. Her wicked sense of humour made tense situations bearable, and she taught me so much. We became collaborators as we were both interested in research, and she became my first paid research assistant. We struggled together to understand the data we were collecting on physiological responses to suctioning through an endotracheal tube in ventilated neonates. We visited a statistician for advice who told us to obtain the mean value for each parameter, this meant we had to count the area (squares) under the curve. We spent hours and hours sitting on the floor in her apartment with reams of graph paper counting the squares to give a mean for heart rate, blood pressure, and respiration. If it wasn't for copious glasses of wine, laughter and jokes we would have gone mad. Today there are software programs that do this automatically, but I will always remember the importance of data and respect those computers that spit out the results. Linda went on the get her PhD in laboratory research, she told me she wanted to give the science back to nursing. Linda became an academic and the first Professor of Neonatal Nursing at the University of Melbourne. She showed that neonatal nurses can be successful academically and remain neonatal nurses. Many others have followed and today when I reflect on these academic pioneers, they strengthen the specialty and its future. They have unique contributions to neonatal nurses and the specialty of neonatal nursing.

During these early days of the specialty of neonatal nursing, two international women stand out, Carole Kenner from the USA and Barbara Weller from the UK. Carole was a diminutive powerhouse of a woman with an outstanding reputation and one of the most brilliant work ethics I have come across. I first met Carole in the early 1990s at a NANN meeting in the US. I was in awe of her as she was the driving force behind neonatal nursing in the USA. She had so much energy and commitment and her vision was to make neonatal nursing visible on the world stage. She was protective of her vision and in 1998 at an international conference on neonatal nursing held in Yorkshire UK, a group of us from Australia and New Zealand put in a bid to bring the International Conference to Sydney in 2000. I had to argue that in Australia we could make a success. I always thought that there was a belief that we were at the end of the Earth and primitive and I was determined to change that view. Over the years I gained her respect as we worked together on the first executive committee for the newly established international organisation (COINN) as it gained international recognition. I have met up with Carole at various events since and we have kept a strong friendship and professional respect.

Barbara Weller from England had impressed me from those early years in London. I knew of Barbara as she had authored a textbook (Baby Surgery) which, for years was the only such book available to nurses who cared for babies following their surgeries. I was in awe of her and when we met I had so many questions for her. Barbara was the editor of the Journal of Neonatal Nursing and was instrumental in helping us set up a similar journal Neonatal, Paediatric and Child Health Nursing in Australia. What I admired about Barbara was her integrity and how she kept her expertise by ensuring set standards were adhered to.

There are many, many more who could be listed here as pioneers, and we are all pioneers in our way. So, why are these pioneers important for the neonatal nurses of today? I think that sometimes the status quo of today is taken for granted without an understanding of why things are the way they are. This applies to the way we do our caregiving to sick newborns and their families as well as the way we work within our profession. Without these pioneering women, we may have been handmaidens to the doctors, working in isolation from other specialty areas, part of paediatrics or even part of midwifery – heaven forbid. There are pioneers today who are forging ahead to acquire new knowledge to support our specialty, changing the way things are done using evidence to support that change, and who are developing a voice for neonatal nursing to inform the wider communities of the work and outcomes of our care practices. Maybe in ten years, I can update these essays with a chapter on these pioneers.

Essay Six

What I have learned from babies

Babies are such interesting beings; the world opens to them with every breath and every vision as they explore their new surroundings. When I was a midwife one of the greatest joys was helping a baby enter the world. When they poked their head out between their mother's legs it was as if they were saying I am here with every cry. It was always emotional for the mothers but also me and always such a privilege and joy. I think in the year when I was helping to deliver babies, I had an adrenaline rush every time. It was like a wow factor.

I often thought that I would have liked to remain a midwife and continue along this continuum of life joining our world. However, I became enthralled by the babies and how they adapted to their strange new world over the first few weeks. I spent hours with them, caring for them and learning about the ways they communicated with their mothers, fathers, and the nurses and doctors. I wondered about the effect of strangers and the babies having to adjust to so many unknown faces. Years later I learned more about this.

So, thinking back now on those early days, what have I learned from the babies? I have learned that each baby is different, they have a very powerful influence on their carers, they are strong, they smell nice, they have potential, and they are vulnerable.

When I first started working with neonates it was during the Paediatric Course. We rotated through various wards and I found the babies and newborns the most interesting.

When they are sick it became more of a challenge. Recently, I found an assignment I had written on a newborn who had a bowel rotation and needed an operation. I surprised myself with the detail of the baby and their responses to the operation and routine things like wound care. I found I could describe their appearance and their behaviour while in hospital, it was like painting a picture with words.

It was a natural progression to become a neonatal nurse, and this occurred initially in London and continued on my return to Sydney. When I became a neonatal nurse and worked closely with babies my learning took off. Thinking back now I remember so many of those babies and what they taught me.

So, what makes me a neonatal nurse? Firstly, it is the knowledge I have gained from study as well as the experience of caring for very small neonates and those with complex anomalies requiring surgery. We all have a catalyst that reminds us of why we are here, what went well and what we can do to improve our care. Lara was my catalyst. She was born at 27 weeks gestation and was admitted to the Neonatal Intensive Care Unit where I was working at the beginning of my career. Lara had difficulty breathing at birth and needed to be on a life support machine (ventilator). I took care of her; she was in an incubator, and I did everything for her to make her outcome as good as possible. This was 40 years ago and when I look at her picture now, I think of my days caring for her and the good and not-so-good. She did make a good recovery eventually and it was very exciting to see her parents take her home. When she was first admitted she was perfect and interestingly her picture shows perfect position and efforts at self-regulation, she had not yet been subjected to intensive care. Her second picture reminds me of why I wanted to continually improve the way Lara was receiving caregiving. Her position looks tortuous lying flat on her tummy with her limbs restricted by heavy splints. Thank goodness we have advanced from these old practices and reverted back to how Lara was when she first arrived. Now we care for babies in a side-lying position, limbs flexed, head in a midline position, and support for the baby to have their hands on their face to help them console themselves. I use these pictures to remind me of the path we (I) have travelled – thank goodness we have cycled back to the beginning – babies teach us this.

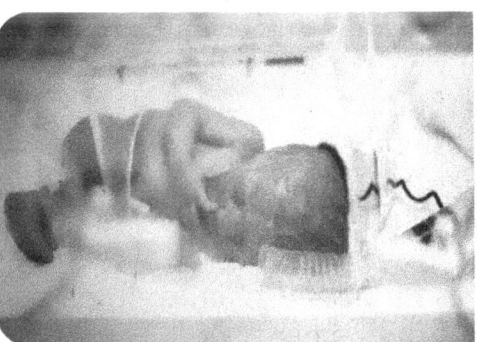 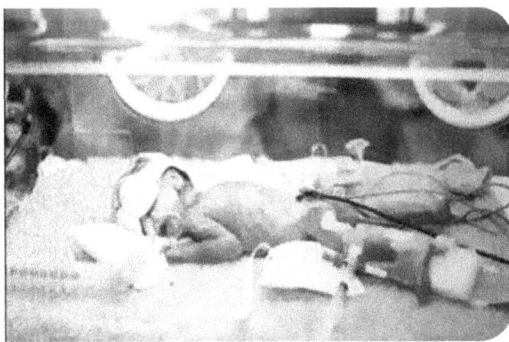

Lara – from perfect to challenging.

What did Lara teach me? Firstly, babies can express pain. In those days there was a fear of using drugs (analgesics) as the side effects were unknown. There was also a myth in those days that if a baby had pain relief, they would need to remain on the breathing machine longer. Lara taught me to be a baby's advocate and part of that was speaking up on medical rounds and pointing out the signs she was showing that indicated pain. I remember with great satisfaction when the team finally agreed, and she was given analgesia and settled. It enabled her to come off the breathing machine earlier. The myths that surround neonatal care sometimes became a block to giving best practices.

Lara's story and others fuelled my interest and eventually my passion to learn more about newborn babies' pain. I studied pain and researched it working on numerous projects to ensure that other nurses were aware of the consequences of babies being in pain. I led a national project to get sucrose as a non-pharmacological pain relief used in all neonatal units across the country, it was so exciting to have nurses in all hospitals working as champions to ensure babies were not subjected to painful procedures without adequate pain relief.

As we gain experience in caring for sick, vulnerable, and very fragile newborns we become vigilant in how we spend our time. Small subtle changes can go unnoticed when nurses are learning or when experienced nurses are busy and that can mean life or death decisions must be made for the neonate. I am a strong believer that we need to spend our time closely watching these babies to prevent stress and deterioration. It does not always work and despite our best intentions, things can go wrong.

For me, the story of David highlights the challenges we face as nurses. David was a twin and, unfortunately, he developed a serious condition of his bowel (necrotising enterocolitis -NEC). He was born very early at 25 weeks gestation and weighed 720grams at birth. He did well for the first two weeks. He was fed tiny amounts of formula milk through a tube into his stomach as his mother was struggling with expressing her milk. He tolerated the formula milk at first but then his abdomen enlarged, and an x-ray showed he had extensive necrosis of the bowel. He went to the operating theatre where the surgeon was only able to save 15cm of his bowel, a very small amount. Despite weeks of being fed through a vein with a special mixture, he was unable to tolerate any milk feeds. David eventually got an infection throughout his body and his reserve just ran out. This was devastating for his family and the team of nurses caring for him. I was an experienced member of the team, and it was a real challenge coming to work knowing that his chances of survival were slim. Eventually, all the doctors, surgeons and nurses came together with the family who decided to offer David palliative care. I found this very challenging because as a neonatal nurse this seemed a contradiction – on the one hand we are caring for babies like David so they can grow and eventually go home but then you must change tack and give comfort care knowing that the baby will die. I worked in the team and had to support the parents as well as the less experienced nurses. Sometimes you ask questions about what went wrong; could the NEC have been prevented; perhaps we should not have given the formula milk feed. So many things could have altered his path. I learned from David and found myself being a strong advocate for breastfeeding and working out ways of supporting mothers so they can express themselves, be less stressed, and eventually produce enough milk to feed their babies. This would reduce the need to use formula milk which we know can contribute to the necrosis.

As I gained more experience, I gravitated toward programs to learn more about the experiences of babies and learn more about their behaviours. The lessons David taught me were that for some babies a better outcome may be death and that helping families come to term with their baby dying and creating memories for them was vital. Things like a scrapbook of his days in the hospital, footprints, cards, helping his mum give him a bath and a cuddle were all part of the care provided. When I get together with my nursing colleagues as a group, we can make it memorable for the families. A neonatal nurse has a very broad and encompassing role. When you care for a baby like David the parents become very respectful of the nurses and the work we do. The parents often ask nurses to attend the funeral when their baby dies. This is extremely hard as you want to support the parents but sometimes it seems to conflict with your professional role. A real dilemma.

Ethics is ever-present in the NICU and there have been many ethical challenges that I have had to think about. The big one is often withdrawal of life support in a baby where life would be either unbearable or painful. These decisions are not easy and often as a nurse, I found myself questioning decisions where nurses are often left to deal with the consequences. In my role, I became very focused and studied caring ethics, so I gained a better understanding of how decisions were made. As part of the team, we would often discuss some of the situations and by having open discussions there was a clearer understanding. Nurses always support parents so when these decisions are made nurses are part of the discussion. Nurses have a unique front-line role and often have the privilege of information shared by the families.

Experience teaches us so much and I have found that, as I became a leader in the field of neonatal nursing, I look back and keep thinking about how we can do things differently, and how we can do better. I found a new passion in developmental care and eventually the Newborn Individualised Developmental Assessment Program (NIDCAP). I found that you can make a difference and, as I learned about the stress of the environment and the impact noise, light and activity have on newborns' sleep and ability to regulate their behaviour I became a champion for a better way of doing things. Now when I look at a small or sick newborn, I find my powers of observation have become finely tuned, not only looking at the heart rate and breathing but the posture, tone, and efforts at self-regulation as well as sleep states. I often think back to Lara all those years ago and if I knew then what now know her time in the NICU may have been of better quality. That is the power of reflection.

I could share stories about my time as a neonatal nurse through the years and sometimes as I scroll through images I think about those babies and how they are doing now. I have seen them when they have returned to the unit for a visit with their parents - you recognise the parents. It is very rewarding to see the outcomes of the care you gave. Sometimes when you see a scar from an infiltrated TPN infusion you gasp, but that is such a small thing when they tell you they have just graduated from high school. I have come to appreciate that following up with the babies who have been in intensive care is so important. We have improved the way we position babies in their cribs based on feedback from the follow-up clinic. A small thing that can make a significant difference. When the babies I have cared for have attended the follow-up clinics you can review their stories and see what can be changed to improve their outcomes, both immediate and long-term.

I am sure every neonatal nurse can think of a few special babies they cared for and the messages they learned. I suggest you hold these memories close as the lessons you have learned will surely help other babies in your care.

Essay Seven

What I have learned from nurses

Recently, I sat in a shared office and had an informal chat with two nurses, Priya and Jeewan who had worked in the NICU for between 10 and 5 years. We talked about neonatal nursing, then neonatology from a historical perspective. The conversation was animated, and I loved sharing my stories with them. What struck me was that they did not know the history of neonatal nursing and even neonatology. This both surprised and concerned me as so many of the practices we do today are built on the foundations of history, and what history has taught us. They were very enthusiastic and had a thirst for any information I could share with them. This made me feel excited and hopeful for the nurses. These essays are a result of this conversation and I thank them for this trigger.

 I would like to share with you a presentation I attended. It was a presentation by three neonatal nurses, Molly a second-year graduate working in the NICU, Amy a nurse practitioner who was endorsed for six months, and Kristen a nurse practitioner who was endorsed 18 months prior. The common theme in their presentation was that their early experiences as students and new graduates in the NICU were a positive experience, not only caring for very complex babies but the support given by their nursing colleagues. Neonatal nurses are a unique group, and we care for each other as well as the babies and their families. If we support our young nurses, then we can ensure our future in neonatal nursing. Not everyone can be a neonatal nurse and as I have travelled and seen neonatal nurses around the globe, we gravitate to each other as we have so much in common, either high tech, primary care, community, or country it doesn't matter as at the heart of our role is that vulnerable neonate.

We learn from each other in many ways. In the early 90s, I travelled to Thredbo in the Snowy Mountains for the Australian Perinatal Society Conference. This was a good meeting as it was the first time an international nurse was invited as a keynote presenter, Linda Bellig, a rather generous woman who was a nurse practitioner from the US. We shared the travel and cars with other nurses heading south as our guest had so many bags from required considerable personal space in our small cars. We drove in a convoy and stopped often for the views and food top-ups! I learned about leadership and how nurses can drive the agenda by being inspirational and articulate on the desired course. Linda gave me a book of stories by nurse leaders - this became my go-to book for inspiration as I embarked on my leadership journey.

Also on this trip was Jo Kent Biggs. I rehearsed my presentation so many times during the four-hour journey that Jo said she could do the presentation. Jo was a special no-nonsense person and was honest with her feedback and opinion. We spoke about how presentations should have a strong message that was inspirational and made others sit up and listen. Every so often someone comes along that you admire, and they know you well and will tell you about your flaws and how to correct them. Jo was one of these people and I miss her honesty. She died too young and has left a legacy as others were also touched by her passion. There is a fine line between work colleagues and friends and my best friends have come from the intimacy of knowing each other through many experiences, both happy and tragic. Jo and I shared many adventures and perhaps the most memorable was our search through Yorkshire for her birth mother. There were highs and lows and our forged bond taught me the importance of friendship. At her funeral, I gave one of the eulogies and it was emotional as well as uplifting to acknowledge such a remarkable friend. Jo taught me that nothing is permanent, and you need to live your life to the fullest as you never know what is around the corner.

Learning takes on all forms and I was always keen to learn all I could about neonatal nursing and the babies in our care. We can get hung up on technology and the medical conditions that infiltrate the neonatal intensive care unit. Nurses continue to amaze me with their expertise and knowledge, and I admire those who have taken the next step and become nurse practitioners. These nurses can straddle the divide between nursing and medicine and keep a nursing focus. However, those early pioneers had challenges keeping a nursing focus as they work on a medical roster. I learned that while nurses are great achievers and have the drive to make a difference, they do need the support of their nursing colleagues.

Nurses are good teachers, and I would like to see myself as a good teacher, mentor, and guide. It is a privilege when a young person seeks you out and wants to follow in your footsteps. I found it flattering when a young student nurse contacted me because she had read about my research on neonatal pain on the internet. I spent some time with her talking about neonates and the challenges they face in the intensive care unit and the many potentially painful things they have to endure. Amy Barker became a neonatal nurse and took on the challenge of understanding newborn pain and how babies can be supported to minimise pain. She also became a researcher and her enquiring mind stood out for me. I enjoyed being her mentor and working with someone with such potential. As a teacher that is one of the most rewarding compliments – to know you helped the career of a young nurse. Since Amy, there have been many more and sometimes I feel like a mother hen proud of her chicks.

I have learned so much from students and more recently I have been a mentor to multiple students undertaking virtual courses. These courses are unique as the students write up their observations of babies through reflecting on their experiences and forward-thinking to care plans and ways to change the system that surrounds the newborn intensive care unit. As each nurse, therapist or doctor open up their thoughts, I feel honoured to be able to share their feelings and frustrations and to be able to guide them to make meaning out of these reflections. I find reflection is such a good way of learning and showing others how you have learned. In a word, I love the reflection, and, in many ways, I am using my reflection in these essays.

Looking back and reflecting on the many nurses I have worked with over the past four decades I get excited as I remember so many good times as well as those challenging experiences. My learning has come from seeking out those individuals who I see as having something to teach me. I would like to take a little time highlighting what you can learn from other nurses, often quiet achievers who are experts in their fields. When I first met Sharon Laing, she was one of those people to whom you are at once drawn. I think it is part personality and part their knowledge of new things. Sharon was a neonatal course student when we met and over the many years, we have become friends. She taught me about perseverance, taking a risk, doing what you felt comfortable doing, and more recent statistics. She is one of those people who has such enthusiasm for life that everything is a joy. Sometimes when I am feeling down, I think of Sharon and her way of exploring ideas and concepts. It gives me sanity, and I do need that from time to time.

Others teach you by being role models with their excellent expertise. One such person is Agneta Kleberg, a Swedish neonatal nurse who I met when I embarked on the NIDCAP training program. Agneta came to Australia and visited several neonatal units in different hospitals. She was calm and polite as she made suggestions for changing practices in the most subtle way you didn't know she was moving you in a new direction. These days when there are so many brash individuals trying to implement change, this calm reassuring nurse taught me a lot. I try to emulate her as I too try to encourage change. I hope I have been successful.

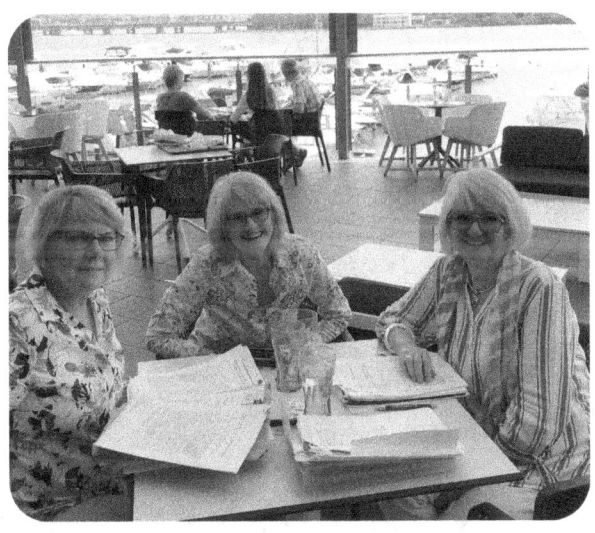

Jann Foster, Sharon Laing and Kaye – making research data fun

Sometimes the friends you make through nursing are unexpected and there is something that gels, and you simply enjoy each other's company. When I first met Joy Browne, it was during the Sydney Olympics when she came to the Children's Hospital at Westmead (the renamed RAHC) to be our NIDCAP trainer. We were wary of her at first as (after all she was an American!) And she has the reputation of being an expert in the field. All a bit scary, however, it turned out she was more in tune with Australians and saw herself as an honorary Aussie. We travelled to many countries together as we taught developmental care and we have laughed so much at many situations. There is something about being in a foreign country where memories just stay with you. Joy and I travelled throughout India sharing the wonder of such a colourful country and being appalled at the level of poverty. We shared a bicycle buggy through the crowded markets of Delhi, ate at dubious roadside huts, and shared the wonder of the Taj Mahal. In South Africa, we went on night-time safaris where a herd of elephants surrounded us, we witnessed a stampede of elephants chasing lions, and lived in accommodation with giraffes and antelope. In the context of teaching developmental care to an audience that was unfamiliar and suddenly the penny dropped, and they understood what we were saying was rewarding. Our road trip through Brittany and Normandy was so memorable with midnight zoom meetings, culminating with a stay on Mont St Michel where we were greeted by a rainbow that summed up our friendship. So, my dear friends, my message is to take the opportunity to get to know your colleagues from far and wide as these are the learning opportunities that stay with you for life.

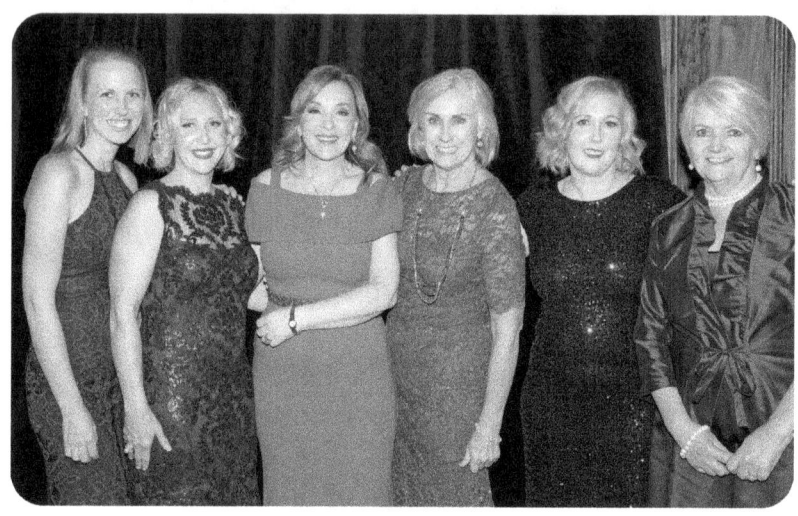

Joy Browne (third from right) with the team from the Australasian NIDCAP Training Centre at a fund-raising event. From left; Kristen James Nunez, Angela Casey, Nadia Badawi, Joy Browne, Nadine Griffiths, and Kaye in 2017

I have been lucky to have learned about neonatal nursing but more importantly, I have learned about life from so many nurses. If I had the last 40 years over again, I think I would have written more about those experiences. Memories are good and reflection kicks those memories into action.

Finally, I would like to mention Julie McNall who left neonatal nursing many years ago but remained committed to babies. During several conversations, I learned through Julie about babies and their personalities. Julie found a way of looking at babies through a different lens and the interconnection between their temperament, behaviour, and views on their world. Finding new ways of 'seeing' babies and looking outside the traditional medical focus can be rewarding and enlightening. My learning is just beginning.

Essay Eight

The birth of a professional organisation

Neonatal nursing became a specialty in Australia in the early 1970s when nurses started to have a voice in many forums. As we met as a group of neonatal nurses, we saw a common need to be united to enable us to have the power to advocate for our specialty which sat precariously between midwifery and paediatrics. These were two strong professional groups that had formed their organisations. Reflecting on my journey with these groups I will not write in chronological order as many events occurred simultaneously. As with any reflections they can become clouded by time, and it is those events that were important to me that have stayed.

Neonatology was becoming well established with doctors training as neonatal specialists. Neonatal Intensive Care Units were expanding and eventually, there were 28 units across Australia. Many of these units were set up as there was a need for the increased survival of premature infants and improvements in obstetrics. With the increase in neonatal beds across the country, the need for highly trained neonatal nurses increased.

Until the mid-1980s neonatal nurses tended to work in the silos created by different intensive care units and the nursing care was predominately directed by the neonatal medical specialists. The neonatal units were mostly staffed by nurses with post-graduate midwifery qualifications as this was seen as an essential qualification to work with neonates. I think this was a remnant of administrators seeing babies as a product of midwifery and obstetrics. Babies were not given individual patient status in many hospitals – a practice that still exists today in some hospitals. Interesting that babies are separate little people but are not given that status to attract individual funding for their hospital stay. I think this extends to other administrative gaps such as a newborn requiring intensive care does not attract funding to adequately provide enough nurses for their 24-hour care. A poor standard I say!

Things began to change for neonatal nursing following the Consensus Conference on the Viability of the Low Birthweight Infants in 1995. This was the catalyst in NSW for the neonatal nurses to get together and form their professional organisation. One of the sessions presented at this forum by Peggy Taylor from Melbourne was "Nursing Workload "and it was the first-time consideration had been given to the nurses staffing the intensive that e care units and the impact of working with these infants at the edge of viability. Peggy put out a challenge to the nurses that they need to have the power to direct their training, lobby for neonatal courses and, of course, have adequate staffing numbers. This call had a profound effect on me and I milled over ways that we could achieve these outcomes. At this time, all the states were different, and Victoria was in the early stages of setting up a professional organisation. We were in no way organised enough to look nationally and thus each state went its own way to become a professional specialty group.

A meeting was held at Royal North Shore Hospital and a group of interested and committed nurses got together. We sat in a circle and debated the current concerns and the future. There was unanimous agreement that we should form a Professional Speciality Organisation. After a lot of finger-pointing and coercion, an executive was appointed and charged with getting the organisation up and running. The name was to be the Association of Neonatal Nurses of NSW, ANN for short. The inaugural executive committee was Jesse Everson as President, me as Secretary, Lynn

Grant as Treasurer, and three members at large Sandie Bredemeyer, Carmel Burton, and Marcia Hampton-Taylor.

The next six months were full of activity. We met at Lynn's flat at Lane Cove in Sydney and spent long hours deciding on the logo, the constitution, and a schedule of meetings. I do have good memories of those meetings with pizza and wine to keep us going. One thing I have to say is that we all agreed, and the meetings were very harmonious. We scheduled meetings around the various hospitals which gave everyone a chance to feel involved. As a way of attracting people to come, we had a guest speaker on most occasions. We felt it was important to keep a clinical focus for the meetings as well as a business meeting to set up the organisation.

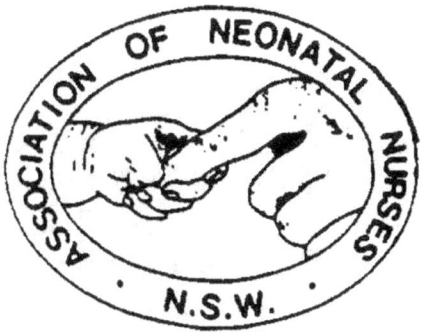

Marcia Hampton Taylor designed the ANN logo

ANN became established and the thing I found most exciting was that it brought together nurses from all the intensive care and special care nurseries across Sydney. We expanded into country areas and the first Country Seminar was held at Coffs Harbour, NSW. Jeanette Walsh, the NUM at Coffs, became our country representative. This link between city and country had an impact on neonatal care as we all began to have an understanding of the challenges facing both country and city. I was lucky to travel across NSW with these seminars and we are grateful to the Rural Medical Service who gave us a plane to fly the committee and speakers to the seminars. It showed how we were seen as filling a gap in the education of the nurses in rural settings. We got to know the pilots who also stayed overnight and joined in the social activities.

When I think back on those early years of ANN there was a great atmosphere of being able to make a difference. The later Presidents of the organisation who were leaders in neonatal nursing in NSW each led the development further and the organisation grew into an influential organisation. Leaders who served as President were Jessie Everson, me, Sandie Bredemeyer, Jo Kent Biggs, Jennifer Dawson, and Jan Nash. There have been others since, but these strong women were the pioneers who forged the history of neonatal nursing in NSW.

ANN was very active between 1989 and 2004. The various committees and workgroups completed many projects and publications. Among these were: a Resuscitation Work package, Neonatal Standards editions 1 and 2, Presentation Guidelines, Guidelines of writing work packages, Research Grants Resource Book, Education scholarship as well as the annual conference and country seminar. There was a lot of activity from dedicated members. The success of these professional groups is dependent on the commitment of the members. We did struggle to bring in a wider group who would be willing to take on some of the project work and take part on the committees. As I look at other groups who have since developed this seems to be a common issue. I loved the work and the friendships that sprung up through working closely together and social activities that enabled us to be seen in a different light. We danced at the dinner functions and were always ready to dress up in various themes. The freedom of expression was rather liberating away from the close focus needed in neonatal nursing.

In these groups, you find like-minded spirits whose company you enjoy. Sandie Bredemeyer and I had the same vision for neonatal nursing and the education pathway for nurses entering the specialty. We submitted position papers with a vision for education, and staffing requirements and championed neonatal nursing at state nursing forums. It was hard but we never gave up. Many years later Sandie told me she was looking for her mojo as she became disillusioned with the health system. We commiserated with each other and gave moral support. It became clear to me that even visionaries need support and sadly the system does not offer rewards to the leaders of change. This is a shortcoming of the current health systems which makes me frustrated as innovation either disappears or goes unrewarded.

Having said that one of my most memorable days was when I was informed that I was to receive an Order of Australia and the following year Sandie also received her medal. We were chuffed as the recognition came from our colleagues and professionals in the specialty of neonatology and perinatology. Not many nurses receive either an AM or OAM, so it was remarkable that two neonatal nurses achieved this honour. I often wonder why nurses are so reluctant to nominate their peers for these honours.

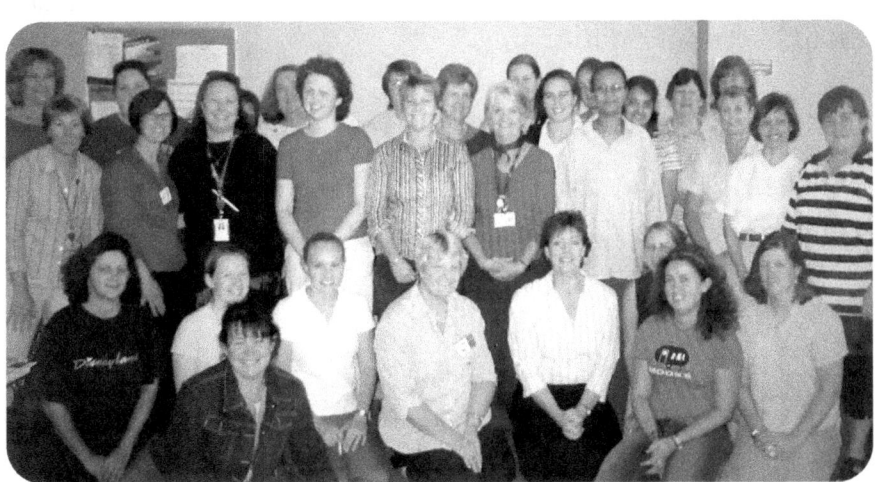

ANN Pow Wow to bring neonatal nurses working in different hospitals together

Simultaneous to the development of ANN in NSW, the other states also set up their own state-based neonatal nursing groups. I need to mention those nurses who led these state groups, Denise Harrison in Victoria (VANN), Trudy Mannix in SA (ANSA), Claire Doherty in Queensland (QNNA), Cheryl Norris in Tasmania (TANN), and Julie Watson in Western Australia (WANNA). This powerful group of women spearheaded the state groups into a national professional organisation.

As we became a global society there was a strong urge to have a national organisation. We had all learned from being influential state groups but there was always the sense that we could be stronger and do more as a national group. There were a lot of preliminary meetings with endless discussions about what national meant. There were still some territories that were not represented and other states struggling to sustain a state organisation. Eventually, we settled on the Northern Territory being represented by South Australia, and the Australian Capital Territory being represented by NSW. Finally, we were able to move forward and look at setting up a national organisation. I took the opportunity to have several meetings with Chuck Rait and Tracy Karp from NANN who offered some sound advice about the constitution and equal representation on the governing board. Advice that was valuable as we went about becoming national.

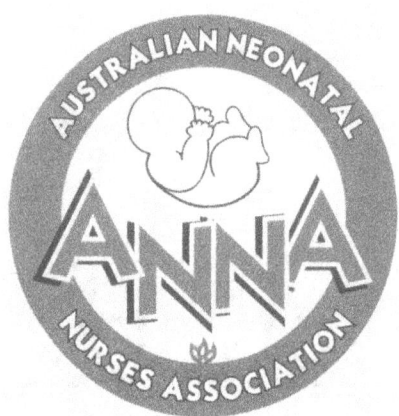

ANNA logo agreed after a competition to find a logo. Won by SA.

The Australian Neonatal Nurses Association is known affectionately as ANNA was born in 1992. We held the landmark meeting at the Australian Perinatal Society annual meeting to allow representation from all states of Australia. I was honoured to be chosen as the first President of ANNA with a representative executive from each state and territory across Australia. What did it mean to be a national group?

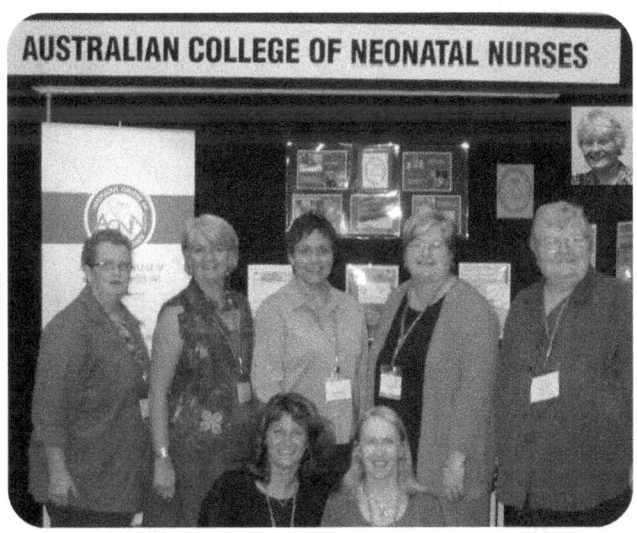

The first eight ANNA Presidents. Back row left to right, Diana Johanson (SA), Kaye Spence (NSW), Vicki Carson (Qld), Julie Watson (WA), Cheryl Norris (Tas). Front, Trudy Mannix (SA), Denise Harrison (Vic). Insert - Sandi Bredemeyer (NSW).

ANNA continued for nearly 10 years before it became the Australian College of Neonatal Nurses. During these years there was a huge amount of change occurring in nursing in Australia. The proliferation of specialty nursing groups led to discussions around credentialing, standards, and competencies in each specialty, the definition of what constitutes a specialty group, and education programs for specialist nurses. Nursing was well established as an undergraduate program and the focus now shifted to post-basic and higher degree programs. To keep abreast of these rapid changes a Professional Officer position was created to inform the executive of the directions ANNA needed to take. I was privileged to become a Professional Officer in 1999.

My term as Professional Officer was one of the busiest roles I have undertaken, and this was purely voluntary, sometimes I asked myself if I really wanted this extra work. I was continually at meetings and national forums where many of these issues were debated. Neonatal nursing was seen as a small specialty area and I was convinced we needed to be part of the debate to get our views heard. While an exhausting role, there was a lot of responsibility attached to it. When I read back over some of the reports I sent, I am amazed at my ability to undertake so much. The role passed to several others who continued to represent ANNA and steer the direction through the maze of nursing developments.

Every national organisation likes to have a forum to enable its members to express their points of view and to encourage the spread of the latest information on the specialty. A newsletter had been produced for years, firstly with ANN then ANNA. This forum did a lot to encourage sharing of information and ideas. However, a Journal was considered necessary to enable members and others to publish their work in a local peer-reviewed journal. The idea for a Journal was championed by Shelly Reid and supported by other experts such as Barbara Weller who was the editor of the JNN – a UK-based journal. I remember her words; "just gather articles and get the first issue out". We were guided by a Journal Management Committee led by Vicki Carson, and we embarked on a joint venture with the NZ Neonatal Nurses and the Paediatric Nurses. The Journal was called Neonatal, Paediatric, and Child Health Nursing. Shelly became the inaugural editor and got the Journal off the ground. The setting-up of this journal was a joint effort and those who should be mentioned are Sandie Bredemeyer and Vicki Carson who did a lot of the leg work to get the journal set up. It was initially slow to request and promote submissions of manuscripts for publication. Cambridge Press in WA was the publisher, and the team was very supportive of our fledgling efforts. Eventually, the journal took off and became the first line of submission for neonatal and paediatric nurses in Australia and New Zealand. I became the second editor when I took on the role in 2004. This was both exciting and terrifying as now I had the responsibility to not only encourage submissions but to work with inexperienced writers to get their work to a publishable standard. What I did learn during my term as Editor was that most nurses cannot write and a lot of time was spent nurturing them to become skilled wordsmiths. Rewarding when you eventually see their manuscripts in print. I was saddened when the Journal ceased publication and to this day I do not understand why. It has left a huge void and our new writers have no local journal to target. For me, it shows a lack of foresight on behalf of the executive, and I hope one day to see the Journal resurrected.

A big turning point for ANNA on the world stage was when we hosted the International Neonatal Nursing Conference in 2001. More on this in another essay. However, ANNA had worked hard to be affiliated with the best. The Perinatal Society of Australia and New Zealand is a large professional organisation made up of basic scientists, obstetricians, midwives, neonatologists, and neonatal nurses along with a smattering of other groups such as therapists, epidemiologists, and consumers. The father of PSANZ was David Henderson-Smart, a neonatologist who I saw as a champion of nurses. He encouraged neonatal nurses to undertake research, and take part in Cochrane Systematic Reviews, something dear to his heart. His passion was the Perinatal Society of Australia and New Zealand (PSANZ) I remember him speaking about PSANZ at the museum in Canberra when they were recording a living history. He was so driven. A goal of his was to have neonatal nurses become Presidents of PSANZ – this was a conversation in a food queue at one Congress and the next thing I knew I was nominated and elected as President. Now that was an interesting four years. It was interesting that anything is possible in a queue and sometimes you can have the best informal conversations in line.

I have been honoured by the ACNN with an honorary Fellowship and PSANZ with life membership. I can't explain how that made me feel, to be recognised by your peers in that way. I was chuffed to say the least and I hope to continue supporting these amazing organisations. Those who have taken on the leadership need the support of the membership as they continue to expand and advocate for neonatal nurses as they support a standard of best practice for newborns and their families.

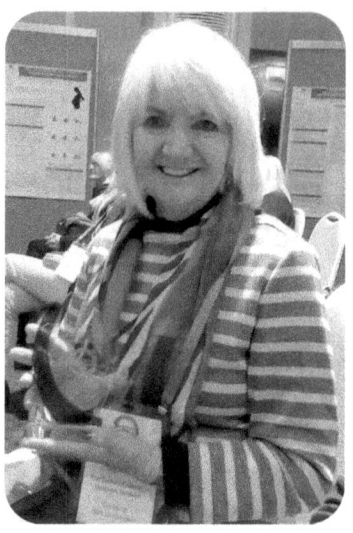

Kaye with her Honorary Fellowship of the ACNN

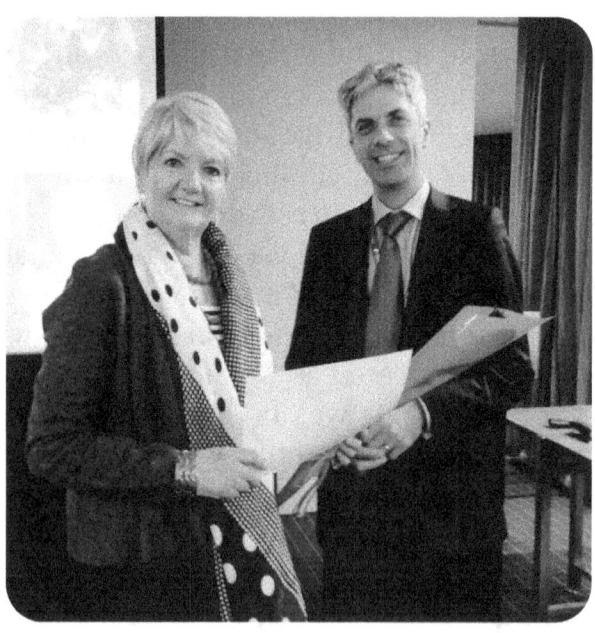

2016 – Kaye presented with honorary life membership of PSANZ by President Frank Bloomfield

Thinking back over the years and my recollections I have recorded here, it was a fantastic journey and my message to the new younger nurses is – if you have the opportunity to volunteer to become involved in a national professional group, go for it, the experience and the comradery are well worth it, and you never know where it will lead. I would not have changed my experiences for anything. The Australian College of Neonatal Nurses has some fantastic leaders, and their vision will lead neonatal nursing into the next decades.

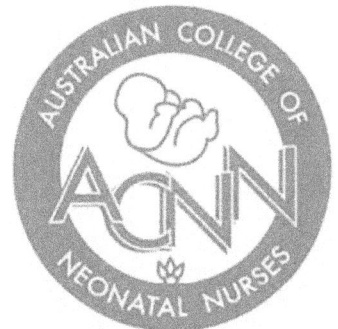

Australian College of Neonatal Nurses logo

Essay Nine

The international stage

There was always the ambition for Australia to host an international conference. A team of Australian and New Zealand neonatal nurses headed to Harrogate in Yorkshire, UK to attend the 3rd International Neonatal Nursing Conference. We had a sneaky motive – to put in a joint bid to host the 4th International Neonatal Nursing Conference. We did a lot of preliminary work and spoke to many people, I guess you could say we lobbied them, about the benefits of holding the next conference in Sydney, Australia. We had done our homework and knew how to woo the Americans and had a budget prepared for the selection committee, which was one person – Carole Kenner.

Harrogate was a historic city, and all the Aussies and Kiwis were dispersed throughout the city in small bed and breakfast hotels. It was so much fun, visiting each other and comparing deals we had achieved. Yorkshire is the home of tea and I remember drinking copious volumes as we met up with old acquaintances and made new friends. A guest at the conference was the Duchess of Kent and we were all dutifully lined up to meet her. She asked me about the Australian cricket team who were touring at that time. Luckily, I followed cricket and could give a sensible answer.

We were successful in our bid and returned home with the prize but a lot of work to do. A committee was formed, a venue chosen, speakers selected, and the program was put together. This conference was a landmark event and put Australia and New Zealand on the international stage. The 4th International Neonatal Nursing Conference was held in

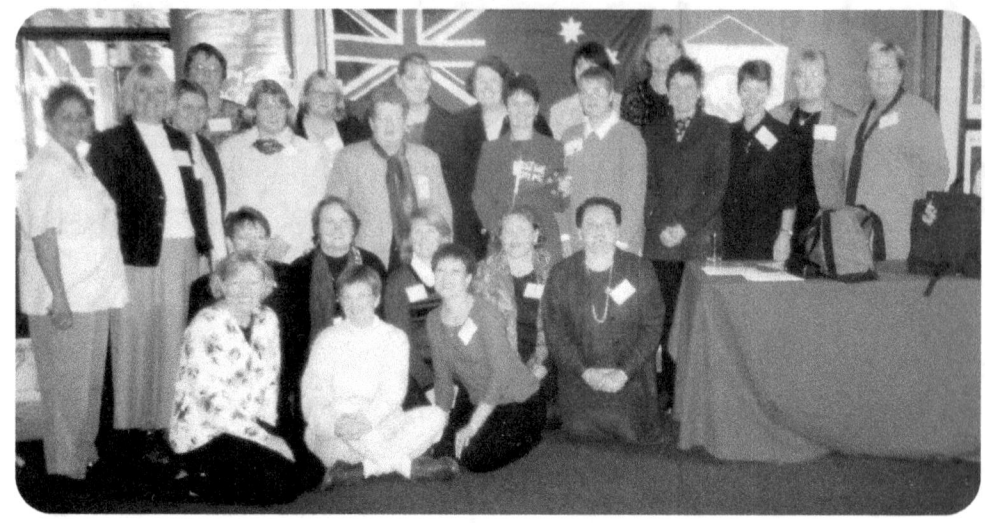

1998 - The Australian and New Zealand delegation at Harrogate, Yorkshire

Sydney in 2001. The conference was a remarkable success and despite 9/11 it went ahead with over 250 international delegates from 18 countries. One of the most memorable events for me was when the 16 nurses from New York and their partners sang their national anthem at the dinner. Normally this would not have an effect on me but as one of those nurses said, "We are so proud to be here, nothing would have kept us away". That showed the determination of neonatal nurses to commit and support each other. I am still in contact with that nurse today – 21 years later. The conference enabled Australian neonatal nurses to highlight their work there were 96 podium and poster presentations. As I look through the names on the program, I see many of the leaders in neonatal nursing today presented at this event. I still get goosebumps when I recall those few days. Since then, there have been 10 international conferences and I hope there will be many more.

A group of international nurses met during the conference to explore the idea of an international federation of neonatal nurses. Carole Kenner presented a paper that led to a lively discussion on how we can become active as an international group. Following on from this meeting a group was convened who met using e-mail to develop a proposal for an international organisation and to set the agenda for progression. These were exciting times as we expanded from Australia and became known in other countries.

The consensus among nurses worldwide was that a global network or international council of neonatal nurses was needed. The purpose of this international group would be to advance global neonatal and maternal health equity. This group was to facilitate educational exchanges with a focus on position statements, standards of care, practice guidelines, and interventions to address the global inequities in neonatal and maternal mortality and morbidity. The plan was for the work to be done through a partnership between developed and developing nations.

In addition to improving worldwide maternal and neonatal medicine and health outcomes, this international coalition was to provide nurses with technical assistance on how best to deliver maternal and neonatal health care services and provide basic state-of-the-art educational and training information to neonatal nurses responsible for delivering health care services, and to situate maternal and neonatal health on the broader policy agenda, globally. Each nation was to develop economic indicators as outcome measures of success. This work would be accomplished by demonstrating the importance of improved health care in economic, social, and educational development efforts worldwide but, most especially, within developing nations. This was a daunting task and a challenge was to spread the work, so it wasn't left to a few willing souls. I was at a crossroads, on the one hand I was keen to be involved as one of the leaders, on the other hand, I was anxious about the commitment and workload. Being something of a workaholic I knew deep down I would be part of the leadership to help spearhead the formation of the council.

The aim was for the group of international nurses to meet and 1) identify the global issues regarding health care equity in neonatal and maternal populations; 2) to solidify linkages among leaders and key personnel from the developed and developing nations to more effectively eradicate the global inequities in maternal and neonatal health; 3) identify specific actions that neonatal nurses globally must take to impact inequities in maternal and neonatal morbidity and mortality; 4) situate maternal and neonatal health in the larger policy arena, especially as it relates to economic, political, social, and educational development within developing nations; 5) engage in strategic planning for working with the International Council of Nurses, the WHO, and other relevant groups, to sustain global efforts to address the inequities in maternal and neonatal health outcomes, as well as identify economic indicators for these outcomes. Grandiose ideas and big words but we were fired up to tackle the task.

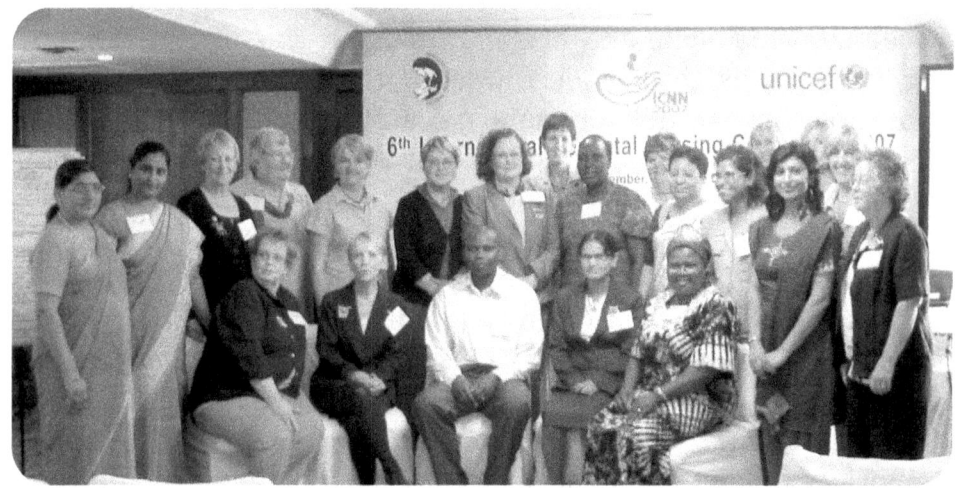

International representations discuss the global network at COINN in India in 2007

The inaugural meeting of this international coalition of nurses was to examine global inequities in maternal and neonatal health outcomes and took place in Ottawa Canada in 2004 at the 5th International Neonatal Nursing Conference. The meeting had approximately 25 key players from around the world who came together to set priorities, objectives and goals. It provided a forum to link maternal and neonatal health to global development efforts. This international coalition of nurses was a small, albeit necessary, step in ensuring the long-term viability of development efforts within every nation. Key members of the steering group were Carole Kenner (USA), Geetha George (India), Ana Quiroga (Argentina), Magda Awases (Zimbabwe), Kaye Spence (Australia), Prissana Soontomchai (Thailand), Noreen Sugrue (USA), Shahirose Premji (Canada). Other participants came from, Singapore, Malaysia, Uruguay, Russia, the UK, Hong Kong, Norway, South Africa, Sweden, Iceland, Nairobi, Finland, New Zealand, Peoples Republic of China, South Korea, and Macedonia. I believe this was a foundation meeting that got us started to consider the needs of nurses to care for babies and families in poor situations. Talking to these nurses was rewarding and certainly gave me insight, I became conscious of just how privileged we are.

These international conferences became essential on my calendar. When I attended the 6th International Neonatal Nursing conference held in New Delhi, India in 2007 I became aware of the magnitude of inequality. This conference introduced me to some of the most gracious and generous people in India. The conference provided a good opportunity to meet up with neonatal nurses from many countries, renew friendships and make new ones. Having attended all five of the conferences gave me a unique perspective to learn about how the different countries managed their challenges.

The conference in Delhi was organised by The National Neonatology (NNF) of India which consists primarily of neonatologists with a few nurses as members. I had the pleasure of getting to know the committee who were a fantastic group of dedicated individuals and, as a collective, put together this really important conference. UNICEF was a co-sponsor which indicated the importance placed on the goals and content of the meeting. Over 900 nurses attended from 30 countries with the majority (750+) coming from India. The audiences were attentive as the enormity of the challenges facing India to reduce the infant mortality rate was the focus of many presentations. Sitting in the large auditorium surrounded by a sea of colourful saris with their wearers attentive to every word spoken. I felt there was a quest and thirst for information and hopefully this newly found knowledge would help the babies and their families.

The pre-conference workshops and sessions were focused on upskilling the nurses from all over India. The workshops were also attended by the international community which enabled many ideas to be shared. I had the pleasure of working with the team from Chandigarh in the day-long workshop – Equipment and Procedures. I was impressed at the preparation that went into the workshop and the dedication of the team in sharing their knowledge and at the same time their thirst for acquiring new knowledge. Dr. Praveen Kumar led the team which consisted of Manjider Kaur, Shakun Oberoi, Karvinder Kaur, Kamlesh Materia, Mabel Rai, and Manpreet Kaur. I learned so much from this team about the challenges facing nurses who strive for best practices in the face of adversity. Things we take for granted are an exceptional challenge for these nurses.

These sessions enabled a sharing of experiences between nurses from many countries and institutions. Sessions were divided into basic and advanced, and it was a challenge to consider ways of interpreting practices in the developed world into the challenges of the developing world. The chairpersons took on the role of moderator to bring the best out of the presenters and to enable discussions and debates. Although challenging to moderate, the results and enthusiasm of the participants was rewarding.

Like all conferences there was an official opening and Renuka Choudhary, Minister of State, Women and Child Development presided. This was an extremely important event as the launch of the Indian Association of Neonatal Nurses took place. This momentous event was the beginning of the recognition of neonatal nursing as a specialty, and it will hopefully have some influence on the retention of the skilled workforce in recognition of the need to have skilled nurses caring for sick newborn infants. This vision was the brainchild of Dr. Manju Vatsa, an exemplary nurse who was an inspiration to all for her dedication and leadership.

The two days of the conference took the audience and presenters on a trip of extremes. The enormity of the challenges facing doctors and nurses in India was overwhelming. Dr. Manju Vatsa described the current scenario of neonatal nursing in India. In the face of the high infant mortality rate and neonatal mortality rate, the focus is on prevention and education. The biggest challenge was the lack of professional status in nursing and the concern about the nursing shortage. The focus was on developing a workforce and training, utilizing, and retraining the nurses. Prakin Suchaxaya from the WHO outlined some priorities such as creating a supportive environment, improving health systems, supporting families, fostering strategic alliances, narrowing the gaps in knowledge, and measuring progress. Interestingly, both developed and developing countries are facing the same issues.

We were treated to a cultural event of classical Indian dancing. The performers took us on a journey of creativity and storytelling. For me, the ultimate experience was while watching the classical Indian dance to the music of Tchaikovsky's Swan Lake. Spellbinding comes to mind. The international delegates contributed to the cultural evening, and I was given the challenge of bringing this together. Everyone embraced the idea, and each country came on stage in turn and 'performed' something from their own country. We had Kenyan singing, Finnish nursery rhymes, and local songs and dance. The Australians sang – 'I still call Australia home' – everyone out of tune! We completed the 'performances' with a Bollywood dance before we were overwhelmed by very enthusiastic local youths joining the dancing!

All conferences have food and often this leads the suggestions on evaluation forms. Nurses love to eat and have variety at conferences. The food was fantastic with delights of the varied cuisine with new tastes and combinations at each meal. The effort that went into making us all welcome was fantastic. The social program enabled us to mix and network in an informal environment accompanied by local entertainment. At the closing Valedictory, I had the honour of representing COINN – the words spoken by various members of the international community will remain with me for a long time to come. Of note were the words by Shela Harani from Pakistan – "I was anxious about travelling so far and leaving my family, I found a new family who made me feel at home." I think this is how many of us felt with the friendliness and warmth of the participants. Many of us took the opportunity to embrace the colourful and comfortable Indian clothing styles and have never been photographed so much! I still have the outfit I bought.

The Council of International Neonatal Nurses then took over the organization of the international neonatal nursing conferences. The 7th International Neonatal Nursing Conference was in Durban, South Africa. The team from New York City said to me after India – "we will be there; nothing will keep us away". That was so true as we met up again in South Africa. South Africa was interesting and again we had many more turn up than we expected. It was as if word got out and everyone came. Local language was a challenge and many of the workshops took place with signs and demonstrations. When I presented with two others – Joy Browne from the USA and Welma Lubbe from SA - our biggest challenge was the technology or should I say the electrical connections. South Africa has vastly different power points and we ended up making connections with a variety of plugs from the USA, Australia, Europe, and the UK and eventually got the projector and computer to work. The lesson I learned from this is to always travel with a selection of plugs and power boards whenever I leave home.

I have enjoyed reliving these events and my travel now includes Belfast Northern Ireland, Edmonton Canada, and Auckland New Zealand as I have followed the international conferences and continue to be amazed at the variety and differences, we have but we share so many other commonalities as neonatal nurses. One memory that stays with me following the International Conference held in Auckland in 2016 was how nurses from many countries were in awe of Heidelise Als the keynote speaker. I got to know Heidi when I became part of the NIDCAP community, and she is an inspirational woman who established developmental care as an important focus for newborn care. To see these nurses watching her and taking every opportunity to meet her was rewarding. Heidi commented to me during an interview I did with her for the Developmental Observer that this was only the second nursing conference that had invited her to present. This took me by surprise but thinking back nurses have been slow to embrace experts from other disciplines.

This leads nicely to my thoughts on the NIDCAP Trainers Meetings which occur each year by invitation. To secure an invitation you need to show your commitment to the NIDCAP (Newborn Individualized Developmental Care Assessment Program) and the associated philosophy of care. As we had a goal to start NIDCAP Training at the Children's Hospital at Westmead in Australia, I was invited to attend. What a revelation this turned out to be. Firstly, the commitment from a wide range of health care professionals, predominately in the USA with a few from the UK and Europe. Interestingly, the trend over the past twenty years has seen a shift in Europe with many countries embracing the training and care.

The first meeting I attended with this group was held in Williamsburg North Carolina. I felt as though I had entered a time warp as this was a historical town set in the 1870s. The Americans take these things very seriously and I could not buy any paracetamol for a persistent headache I developed. The rationale: they didn't have these drugs in 1870! Apart from that, I had become the target of a fanatic who I shared a car with from the airport to the hotel. She was not part of our group, but she would put sheets of the information under my door each night on the holocaust. Why? Well, I made the mistake of not keeping my mouth shut and mentioned that Australia was sympathetic to the Palestinians. I learned my lesson and now I try not to engage in hot topics with strangers. At this first NIDCAP meeting,

I became acutely aware of the hierarchy of the NIDCAP Federation International (NFI). I met some interesting leaders in this movement and today individuals such as Inga Warren from the UK, Jacques Sizun from France and Bjorn Westrup from Sweden remain key people I admire for their passion and commitment.

I have attended a dozen meetings since this first one. These have been great as I have been afforded the opportunity to travel to so many countries and experience some amazing speakers. I have found these meetings inspiring and I loved the networking that occurs with health professionals and families from all over the world. At the first meeting, I was told I was very brave to ask questions and challenge some of the presenters. This was strange for me as all my career I felt comfortable speaking up and challenging some of the ideas presented. Maybe I was one of those people whose opinions needed to be heard!

The global collaborations that stemmed from these meetings have given me opportunities for sharing ideas and innovations. When the Grace Centre for Newborn Intensive Care was credited with being a NIDCAP Training Centre I felt an ambition that rose in the late 1990s had finally come true. The Australasian NIDCAP Training Centre has become an established focus for many NIDCAP Training Centres, and I admire nurses who have taken on the challenging roles associated with the Centre.

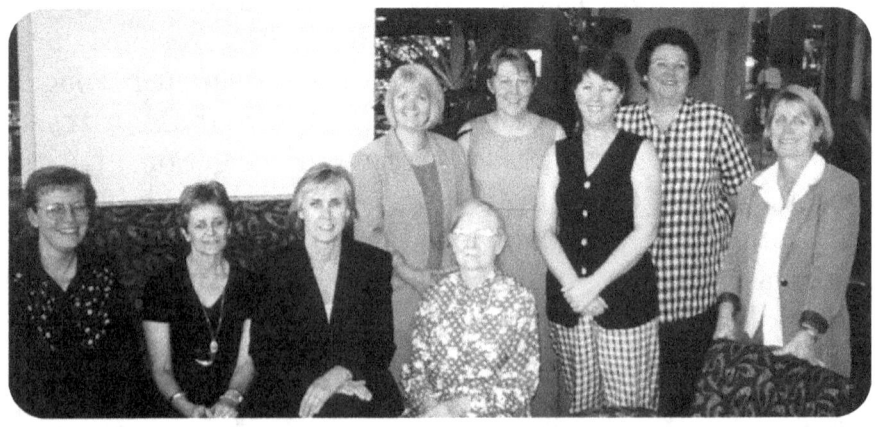

The original group of NIDCAP Trainees in Grace Centre for Newborn Intensive Care – 2000

Nadine Griffiths became the first NIDCAP Trainer in Australia and has taken the Centre from strength to strength. When I first met Nadine, it was through clinical supervision; she wanted a mentor who would challenge her in her professional development. Little did she know I had targeted her to move into neonatal nursing and eventually take on NIDCAP. Sometimes when you see potential you just must make that potential work for you. In this case, it was a success.

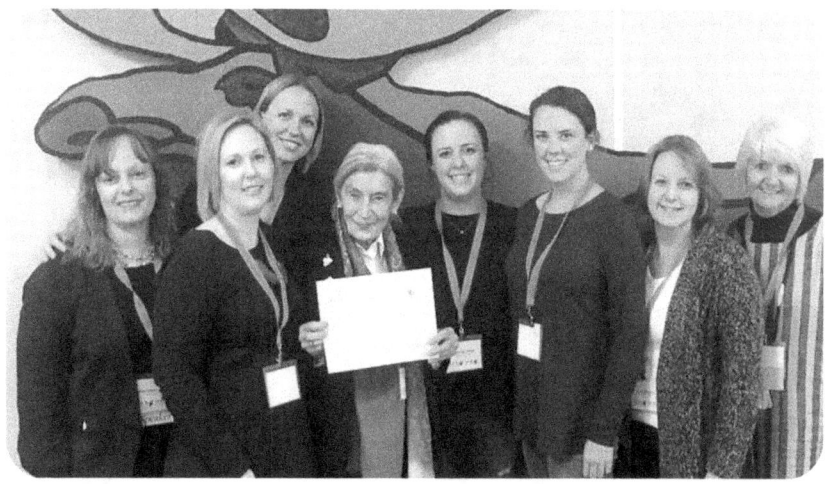

Australasian NIDCAP Training Centre receiving certification from Dr Heidelise Als in Edmonton, Canada

Thinking about the international scene, it is still important for neonatal nurses in Australia to be aware of the issues confronting nurses in other countries. It puts into perspective our issues and the resources that are available. ANNA has spread to some developing countries through special interest groups that take on the task of teaching nurses in New Guinea. This sharing of information and seeing the issues firsthand can help nurses prove their priorities by being aware of the enormity of the challenges facing our peers in other countries.

Essay Ten

Researching and publishing

Every specialty is driven by research to do things better and to share its findings with others both locally and globally. I found as I progressed through my career in neonatal nursing, that research took hold, and I was fascinated with the questions that arose from clinical practice. I have found many nurses are afraid or scared of research and tend to leave it to others to find the answers. I often used a cartoon that showed nurses running away from research. There are nurse pioneers who have led research and made it accessible to others. I would like to think of myself as one of those nurses.

Nurse researchers are different from research nurses. The former has the inquiry to improve nursing practice. They lead research, and understand the rigor needed, they learn about data management, analysis, and writing up and disseminating their findings. In my time, I have worked with some outstanding nurse researchers and specifically neonatal nurse researchers. They often love to teach and look to those individuals who show potential. They also know when to collaborate and use the skills of others to enable them to complete their research.

When I started in neonatal nursing, research was far from my agenda. I wanted to be an excellent clinical nurse and only slowly moved into teaching and education. This seemed like a natural progression for an experienced and senior neonatal nurse. Clinical teaching opened up my interest in research as I sought out the evidence to support my teaching. When I became a clinical nurse consultant, research was one of the five domains of our practice. The research was still elusive to many in these roles, and I became determined to make research interesting and even exciting for clinical nurses. This was no easy feat. Many nurses think research is statistics and tended to shy away.

Thinking back over the years. the nurse researchers who made their mark on neonatal nursing are ones I admire for their bold venture into research. Linda Johnston who I have previously mentioned did science and lab research for her PhD so she could put her knowledge back into neonatal nursing. I have never forgotten those words, though she probably has. Linda was a data collector for a study on nursing workload and patient acuity in the early 1990s. Interestingly we are still gathering data for this topic 30 years later. One thing nurses tend not to do is use the evidence from research to improve their working practices. I was a lead researcher for another workload study, the same topic, same population, and nurses would not use the findings. This still baffles me today and one thing I wanted to make sure happened before I retired from neonatal nursing was to ensure we had some measures of nurses' workload to be able to decide if experience and patient acuity makes a difference. I maybe still waiting when I go to my grave!

Other brilliant neonatal nurse researchers continue to drive research. Sharon Laing who has a knack for making statistics interesting and more importantly getting nurses to understand them. Sharon is a good friend, and I am continually inspired by her enthusiasm as she continually learns and shares her new knowledge. She has a sense of humour which goes a long way in shaping the future path for nurse researchers. Another student from the neonatal course who went on to be a leader in research was Deborah Harris who is now in New Zealand. Deborah has shown the world how to be a good collaborator and has made some ground-breaking changes for babies with hypoglycaemia and low blood sugars. Deborah has shown me a passion for research and the need to be continually striving for best practice. Some other nurse researchers I met through collaborative research and Jann Foster falls into this group. I was involved in a study with Jennifer Greenwood, a diminutive but powerful nurse who taught me so much about researching nurses. She too had a sense of humour and now I think that is a necessity for a nurse researcher. Jann, a neonatal nurse, was Jennifer's research assistant and together we were challenged to theme recorded transcripts of nurses' thoughts as they did their patient caregiving. We spent hours deliberating over the meaning of the transcripts and even today I think about the language of nurses and the jargon used. Jann now teaches at a university and has the strongest commitment to research and evidence I have come across. I feel the students are in good hands to be taught about research by her. Her most memorable session was getting nurses to think about research design was by getting them to decide which shoes to buy. This innovation is typical and shows how creative nurses are.

Of course, there are so many nurses who have taken on the commitment to research and have made or are soon to make their mark in research. Some names that come to mind are; Carmel Collins, Sandie Bredemeyer, Margo Pritchard, Denise Harrison, Mary Lou Morritt, and Margaret Broom amongst others. I feel if nurses are allowed an opportunity to experience being part of the research process they will develop an appreciation or even excitement about research. I had this vision in the mid-2000s and set about setting up a fellowship program for clinical nurses to learn about research and undertake a small research study. Looking back now I can see the success of the program and the eight nurses who completed the program. It is such a reward for me. I can see how they have made a contribution and I feel comfortable knowing that there are nurses who will take up the baton for neonatal nursing research. Thank you, Amy Barker, Kristen James Nunez, and Jeewan Jyoti.

The ACNN now has a Research Special Interest Group where like-minded nurses meet and talk about research and promote their interests among their peers. This group was first set up by Shelly Reid who handed it over to Margaret

Broom in recent years. The camaraderie and support among this group highlight to me how networking is beneficial for all and especially the babies, families, and nurses who are the recipients of the best practice based on current evidence.

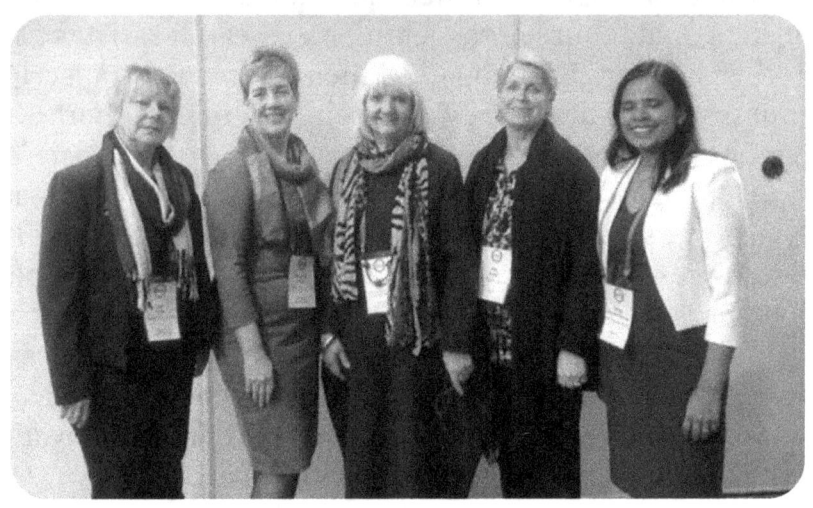

ACNN Research Special Interest Group – Jann Foster, Margaret Broom, Kaye, Kim Psaila and Sheeja Pathlore

Of course, when we talk about research, we also need to put it into the context of sharing the findings. The best way is to present at a conference and then follow this up with a publication. However, this has been poorly practiced as many nurses either cannot write or are afraid of the rigour and possible rejection from publishers. Something which I believe can be overcome. For nurses to be able to publish there needs to be a journal that is encouraging and enables submissions to be supported. ANNA was a third of the new Journal named Neonatal, Paediatric, and Child Health Nursing, and Shelly Reid was the inaugural editor.

Thinking back to my own journey to become published, it was certainly a hard slog. My first publication was a joint effort to write up a case study on congenital diaphragmatic hernia which was published in The Lamp. They took clinical articles back in the mid-90s. It was amazing, I hand drew a picture as I could not find one to use in the publication. It also won a prize. A pretty good start and it certainly gave me the confidence to start sending more articles for publication. I wish all new authors had this experience. Of course, it didn't last, and I soon became familiar with rejection. What I have learned is to make sure you list potential reviewers who are sympathetic to your topic. As a reviewer now for many journals I consider it an honour to review someone's research work and I make sure my feedback is meaningful, thoughtful, and helpful.

Unfortunately, due to reasons I still find hard to understand, the NPCH Nursing journal ceased to exist. The governing committee of the ACNN decided not to renew the contract with Cambridge Media and try for a more international publisher – the result was the demise of the journal. As I discuss publication with novice nurse researchers it is hard to find a suitable journal for their inaugural submission. It is sorely missed and, I hope one day we will again have a specialty journal available in Australia.

Many years ago, I wrote an editorial titled 'Why Nurses Should Write'. In this piece I focussed on the need to share our experiences and what we have learned from being neonatal nurses. Neonatal nurses have a lot of information to share and by writing up case studies it adds to the body of evidence for neonatal nursing. Writing does not have to be research driven, but it needs to be good. This is where collaboration with nurse academics or those with an experienced track record for publications can help. Of course, those nurses doing research have an obligation to write and publish their findings. Too often nurses are choosing to undertake quality improvement projects with adequate supervision, and these may get rejected due to a lack of rigor in the project. Experienced nurse leaders have a responsibility to ensure we have a sound body of evidence for what we do. Recently the ACNN partly funded a study to show nurse-sensitive outcomes of neonatal nursing. I look forward to seeing the results of this study as it may be a way forward to ensuring neonatal units are adequately staffed.

Essay Eleven

Those who influenced me

Reflection is a powerful tool to enable us to see the building blocks that helped us get to where we are today. In Neonatal nursing, there have been so many people who have contributed to the development of the profession. Many of these influential persons have left a lasting impression on various members of the profession. Often it is the unassuming individuals who strive for their achievements and who have contributed to the development of the profession. These individuals coupled with the changes that have occurred in Neonatal care over the decades form our history. I believe we need to keep, acknowledge and enshrine our history for our future generations. Speaking to some of our newer nurses about their goals and aspirations for Neonatal nursing has inspired me to ensure they know the history and why we work as we do today.

During my 45-year career in neonatal nursing, so many people have left their impressions on me, and I believe have helped me to become the leader I am in neonatal nursing. I would like to share these 'influencers' with you and, hopefully, reading about these individuals will make you think of those who have influenced your careers. The following paragraphs are in no particular order but as they came to mind.

David Henderson Smart. David was affectionately known as DHS to most people and he held a special place in the hearts and minds of many neonatal nurses. DHS was a neonatologist and Professor of Perinatal Medicine at Royal Prince Alfred Hospital. My early memory of DHS was when he was the Cardiac Fellow at the Royal Alexandra Hospital for Children at Camperdown. He had an air of authority but was one of the fairest people I knew. He acknowledged the contributions from all levels of health professionals and, he had a passion for evidence. I had the pleasure of working with DHS on many committees and working groups. The most influential for me was on the Perinatal Committee which was a Ministerial appointed committee that arose from the Shearman Report into Maternity Services in NSW. I was privileged to be one of two appointed nurses to this highly influential committee, the other nurse was Heather Mann from Newcastle. Sometimes I was fearful of saying the wrong thing and of making a mistake as I argued for the nurses' view on the re-organisation of Perinatal Service across NSW. DHS always acknowledged our opinion and was supportive of some of the more controversial decisions made. He taught me to stick with my opinion, often in the face of objections from others. Later in the early 20s I worked with DHS on a national project to close the evidence gap for pain in newborn infants in the hospital. This was to be DHS's last project and publication before his untimely death. Working closely with him for almost two years I learned from the master. I watched him negotiate with many doctors and administrators and I saw him become frustrated when there was a lack of response. He has influenced the way I see adversity and has set the bar high for ensuring excellence in clinical practice. He was so excited when he told me he had been made an honorary member of the Australian College of Midwives, something he always held close. My fondest memory of him was in Canberra at the new Contemporary Museum during one of the Perinatal Society of Australia and New Zealand (PSANZ) conferences There was a room set up for Australians to record their messages to be kept for posterity. DHS spoke on his passion for newborn care, keeping mothers and babies together and, most of all, the professional multidisciplinary organisation. He was so proud of the work and how all health care professionals, scientists and families work together. I think this influenced me more than I knew at the time and my passion for neonatal nursing and the Australian College of Neonatal Nurses could rival his.

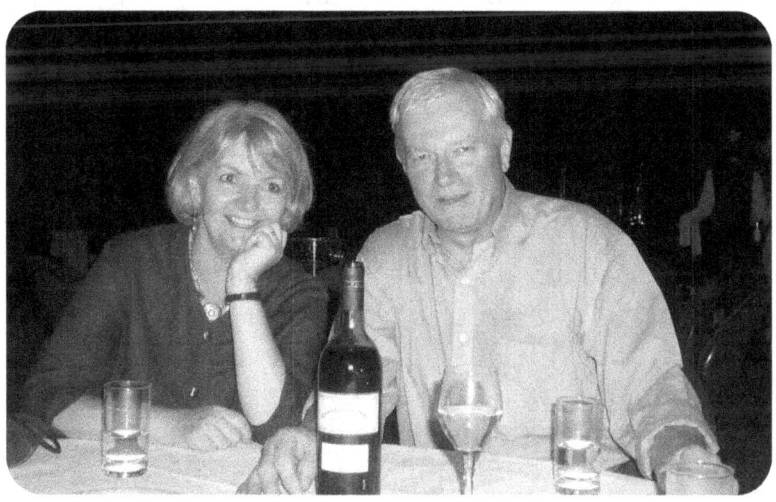

1996 – Kaye with David Henderson Smart at PSANZ dinner

Anthea Blake. Anthea was the charge nurse in the neonatal unit at University College Hospital in London. I first met Anthea when I started at UCH to do the Neonatal Intensive Care Course. What struck me about Anthea was the knowledge and skills which she never promoted. She quietly went about her work and would weave her way through the nursery adjusting positions, tipping water out of CPAP circuits, and answering the most mundane questions all while leading the rounds of her medical colleagues. She showed me what multi-skilling was and how a roving eye can pick up insignificant things before they become big problems. Everyone, from the most junior nursery nurse to the Professor of Neonatology bowed to her ability and her quiet unassuming way of running a neonatal unit. I have tried to emulate her throughout my career and how I would have liked to meet up with her again when I became a leader, just to give her some feedback. We are never really good at that .

Andrew Berry. Andrew is one of those people who had a vision and did not give up until that vision was achieved. He was a Neonatal fellow in Baxter Ward at the Royal Alexandra Hospital for Children in Sydney when I returned to Australia after working in London for ten years. He was soon appointed a Staff Specialist in Neonatology. I remember we decorated with ribbons the incubator of the first baby admitted under his care. He was humble in his acknowledgment, and I think it showed how popular he was with the staff. Andrew went on to set up the state-wide newborn transport team and the establishment of NETS. What influenced me about his vision was his recognition of nurses as part of the retrieval team and ultimately having nurse-led retrieval teams. If you have a vision you need to stick with it even when there is adversity to the process. His attention to detail is one of the biggest influences I remember. He knew the equipment minutely, the protocols by heart, and how to circumnavigate administrators, with a calmness that almost made you unaware of what was happening. He had a pilot's license and flew his plane often to conferences, offering a seat to us nurses as a fare-saving venture. I remember meeting him at Bankstown Aerodrome with 3 others heading to Launceston for the PSANZ Conference. He spent some time with a technician or engineer discussing some repairs that had to be done. During the flight, we asked what the 'technical' problem was, and he calmly said the mice had eaten through the cables. He said not to worry it was all fixed, the only problem was they didn't find the mice! We cautiously sat in the plane watching the floor for evidence of mice. It was only during a break at Moruya that we saw the twinkle in his eye and the joke he had on us. That was typical of Andrew and his influence on me extends to keeping a lighter side to problems.

Madge Buus Franck. Madge is a nurse practitioner from Dartmouth in the USA. I first met Madge at an International Neonatal Nursing Conference in Canada. I knew of her through her many publications and reputation through NANN, the American neonatal nursing organization. Madge was one of those people you admire for their ability and her people skills. She had an amazing ability for making friends and bringing people together from many distinct groups. In India, I was influenced by the way she sought out the quiet and shy local nurses who must have felt estranged from all the foreign nurses competing for attention. Everywhere I looked I would find Madge surrounded by maybe 6-8 nurses and she was speaking and laughing with them in a relaxed way. What she learned from them was unique and her experience at the conference was so different from most of the nurses from other countries. Madge's influence has remained, and I find when I am at a conference, either international or local I try to emulate her and bring together nurses (or delegates) who may be attending their first conference, or who are shy and alone in their attendance.

Vicki Carson. Vicki is one of those no-nonsense people who command respect. Vicki and I worked together on the NPCHN Journal. I was the editor, she chaired the Journal Management Committee, and her mother, Valmay, was my editorial assistant. Vicki worked at Townsville Neonatal Unit and became the Nurse Manager and has since climbed into the Executive Directors Position for Women and Newborn Services. What I like about Vicki are her people skills and a wicked sense of humour. Vicky is one of the best administrators I have come across and what makes her unique is that she has not lost touch with her beginnings as a neonatal nurse. She served a term as President of ANNA and held a vision for neonatal nursing that matched mine. Vicki's influence on me stems from her knowledge of the system and how to progress your plans to make sure you achieve what you want. I recently drew on Vicki's ability for a review I was undertaking. I knew she could provide me with the information I needed and, her generosity of time and knowledge has influenced the way I work with people. I like to think that helping nurses in new positions can ultimately achieve my goal, to see a strengthened neonatal nursing profession. I value Vicki's friendship and the honest feedback she is prepared to share.

Joy Browne. I had a vision that I would like the Grace Centre for Newborn Care to become a NIDCAP Training Centre. Part of this vision was to have NIDCAP in Australia and developmental care as the focal model of care for newborn infants across all neonatal units in all states. Joy Browne, from Colorado in the USA, was able to influence me to achieve this vision. Joy is a very skilled NIDCAP Trainer and a respected member of the international NIDCAP community. I have known Joy over the past 20 years, and her honesty about my vision and how to go about achieving it has influenced me to become actively involved in the NIDCAP Community. There is something special about some colleagues and how they tend to morph into friends. This is what happened between Joy and me and, as I got to know her more, I realised her influence was starting to have a profound effect on me. I could see past barriers, the road ahead became clearer, and I saw the vision ahead. Joy not only influenced me, but she was also quite the manipulator. She took on the role as my campaign manager when I stood for the NIDCAP Federation International board of directors, I might add she influenced me to take on the nomination. I learned so much from this experience and will always be grateful. We have travelled together in India, South Africa, and France, and the influence of a fellow traveller in new and unexpected places can take on a new focus. I respect her and she revels in the fact she is an honorary Aussie.

While I have named and described a few influencers in my neonatal career there are many more. Some are nameless as I can only remember certain instances, others have influenced me in subtle ways, and still, continue to influence me. Those listed here have each offered a unique influence on me and have contributed to the neonatal nurse I became and remain today. I would like to think the influence of these individuals has spilled over into my personal life and as I move to retirement, I will continue to value their influence.

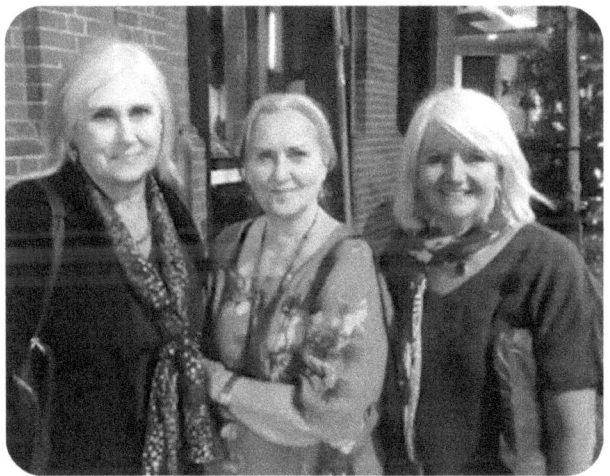

2017 – Joy Browne, Julie McNall, and Kaye. Networking and social interaction.

Essay Twelve

A crystal ball to the future

I titled this collection of essays – Looking Back to See the Road Ahead. What is the road ahead? For me, as I move towards retirement, there are some who say I will never retire, that road ahead is something I want to travel as I take on a different challenge. I will however always remain a neonatal nurse and will hopefully continue to use the skills and knowledge I have gotten from a long and rewarding career.

So, what now for the profession of neonatal nursing and the professional organisation that supports it? When I look into the crystal ball of the future, I see some good things, but I also see many challenges.

Looking back over the years, neonatal nursing has developed into a specialty built on knowledge, skills, and evidence for practice. Babies and their families are cared for in a humane way where the individual infant and their family are respected for their wishes, differences, and individuality. Comfort and a stress-free environment are paramount and, nurses will challenge the health care team to ensure this occurs.

For the past twenty years, I have worked towards a vision of setting up a NIDCAP Training Centre in Australia. That vision became a reality in 2017 when the Australasian NIDCAP Training Centre was certified by the NIDCAP Federation International in the Grace Centre for Newborn Intensive care. I know this will make a difference to the babies and their families as nurses, doctors and, allied health professionals take on the responsibility for implementing individualised developmentally supportive care. This focus is part of the initiative of the first 2000 days of a child's life, from conception to two years of age, which is an important foundational period that shapes their development and wellbeing. Reducing stress supports the development of the brain during this vulnerable period, positively influencing employment, health and, relationship outcomes for the rest of their lives. To know that the care provided will contribute to these outcomes is rewarding. I am reminded again of Lara and the environmental stress she experienced. NIDCAP (Newborn Individualised Developmental Care Assessment Program) is brain protection for premature and critically ill newborns. The program teaches nurses and allied health professionals as well as parents, how to support these fragile babies and, teaches strategies to reduce noise and light to protect sleep and comfort measures during painful procedures. We have come so far, and I find it comforting to know that my vision has become a reality.

There have been advances in the treatment of complex conditions. Technology is more refined however, there is a need to consider its use rather than just use it. Drugs have made it easier to treat specific and complex conditions and we are more aware of potential side effects and the impact on long-term outcomes. Many years ago, there was talk of an artificial womb, this is now a reality as we mimic foetal positioning, changes to the environment through modifying the light and sounds and paying attention to hydration and skin care. So, my crystal ball tells me this will continue to improve and as we learn more from the babies and research, we can hopefully reduce unwanted effects and poor outcomes.

Nurses continue to be a valued service and having a well-staffed and educated neonatal nursing workforce still is an important goal. However, I despair at the thought that the struggle will continue. We have been continually striving for tools that will enable us to say we need a certain number of nurses to care for a certain number of babies at a certain level of acuity. Nurses need to be skilled to be able to care for high acuity and vulnerable newborns and they need to be critical thinkers and decision-makers who collaborate with the medical and allied health teams. I look ahead into my crystal ball and, I do not see this goal. Neonatal nurses will have to become more political and campaign for the number of skilled nurses to enable them to supply a high level of care. Instead of being punished for speaking out, nurses should be applauded and supported in their quest to achieve best practices for the most vulnerable of patients and afford them the best outcome possible. After all newborn infants are our future, society's future.

The specialty of neonatology and neonatal nursing has many challenges ahead. Being a small highly specialised group, it is still difficult to influence decision-makers and administrators. I see a threat of amalgamation from Paediatrics as they move to incorporate this highly motivated and emotive group. The Australian College of Neonatal Nurses needs to remain strong and astute to these threats and support the membership as they strive to achieve their goals. Neonatal nurses need to inform the community, administrators, and politicians about what they do, what makes them unique, and what makes them needed.

Recently I have met some truly inspiring nurses working across many hospitals in Australia. I have confidence that these nurses will become the next leaders in the profession of neonatal nursing. This looks good for the future. So, as I look back, I have seen my path ahead and I leave knowing newborns and their families are in good hands.

Epilogue

I have enjoyed the experience of writing from memory and sharing what I consider to be the salient events in the development of neonatal nursing across Australia.

I have set the date for my retirement, and it will be interesting to see if I do commit to this date.

Some of the activities I will continue for the time being are:

Senior Editor for the Developmental Observer, this will enable me to continue to contribute to NIDCAP, a passion I acquired in the last two decades. It will also allow me to continue encouraging submissions from across the globe and to provide a truly international focus.

Casual mentor the FINE 2 Program. Later in my career I found this program inspirational. One reason is that it uses reflection as a learning tool. I have gotten so much from the student's assignments, and I love reading them and seeing the babies and their families through their eyes and descriptions of their observations.

Member of the supervision team for Nadine Griffiths' PhD. I believe in the study Nadine is undertaking and I am committed to seeing it through. Nadine is inspirational in the way she thinks about the babies and how she uses every bit of technology in her approach. When Nadine obtains her PhD the knowledge, she will share will be vital to the further development of developmental care education.

Mentor by request. I have a passion for nursing and neonatal nursing and would like to encourage nurses as they work their way through their careers. Happy to have casual conversations, afternoon teas, lunches, and drinks.

Pursue my creative writing, revisit Paris my writing inspiration, revise my webpage (**http://kathrynkaye.com.au**) and have my books published. I have chosen creative writing as a way to continue my personal growth through imagination, memories, research, and fact-finding. I love the fact that I can create stories from all realms, even contradictory to science.

I am and will always be a neonatal nurse and as I move onto a new chapter, I am proud of the team I leave. An honour was bestowed recently with the launch of the Kaye Spence AM scholarship. I hope the nurses who receive this scholarship are inspired to contribute to neonatal nursing. It can only go from strength to strength with our future leaders.

www.ingramcontent.com/pod-product-compliance
Lightning Source LLC
Chambersburg PA
CBHW050300120526
44590CB00016B/2432